Racial Sensitivity and Multicultural Training

Recent Titles in
Contributions in Psychology

Soviet and American Psychology During World War II
Albert R. Gilgen, Carol K. Gilgen, Vera A. Koltsova, and Yuri N. Oleinik

Counseling the Inupiat Eskimo
Catherine Swan Reimer

Culturally Competent Family Therapy: A General Model
Shlomo Ariel

The Hyphenated American: The Hidden Injuries of Culture
John C. Papajohn

Brief Treatments for the Traumatized: A Project of the Green Cross Foundation
Charles R. Figley, editor

Counseling Refugees: A Psychosocial Approach to Innovative Multicultural Interventions
Fred Bemak, Rita Chi-Ying Chung, and Paul B. Pedersen

Health Related Counseling with Families of Diverse Cultures: Family, Health, and Cultural Competencies
Ruth P. Cox

Acculturation and Psychological Adaptation
Vanessa Smith Castro

Progress in Asian Social Psychology: Conceptual and Empirical Contributions
Kuo-Shu Yang, Kwang-Kuo Hwang, Paul B. Pedersen, Ikuo Daibo, editors

Vygotsky's and Leontiev's Holographic Semiotics and Psycholinguistics: Applications for Education, Second Language Acquisition and Theories of Language
Dorothy Robbins

The Arts in Contemporary Healing
Irma Dosamantes-Beaudry

The Politics of Stereotype: Psychology and Affirmative Action
Moises F. Salinas

RACIAL SENSITIVITY AND MULTICULTURAL TRAINING

Martin Strous

Contributions in Psychology, Number 46
Paul Pedersen, Series Adviser

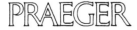

Westport, Connecticut
London

Library of Congress Cataloging-in-Publication Data

Strous, Martin.
    Racial sensitivity and multicultural training / Martin Strous.
       p.   cm.—(Contributions in psychology, ISSN 0736–2714 ; no. 46)
    Includes bibliographical references and index.
    ISBN 0–275–98148–7 (alk. paper)
    1. Psychiatry—Social aspects—South Africa. 2. Mental health services—Social aspects—South Africa. 3. Racism—South Africa—Psychological aspects. 4. Apartheid—South Africa—Psychological aspects. 5. Cultural psychiatry—South Africa. 6. Ethnopsychology—South Africa. 7. South Africa—Race relations—Psychological aspects.
    I. Title. II. Series.
    RC451.S6S776   2003
    362.2′042′0968—dc21   2003053557

British Library Cataloguing in Publication Data is available.

Library of Congress Catalog Card Number: 2003053557
ISBN: 0–275–98148–7
ISSN: 0736–2714

First published in 2003

Praeger Publishers, 88 Post Road West, Westport, CT 06881
An imprint of Greenwood Publishing Group, Inc.
www.praeger.com

Printed in the United States of America

The paper used in this book complies with the
Permanent Paper Standard issued by the National
Information Standards Organization (Z39.48–1984).

10 9 8 7 6 5 4 3 2 1

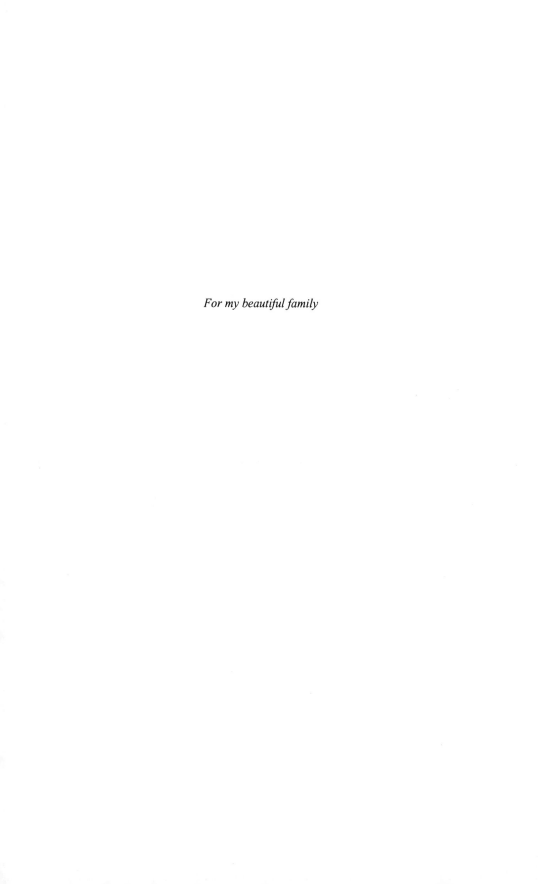

For my beautiful family

Contents

Series Foreword

Paul Pedersen

We can perhaps learn more from our mistakes than we can from our success. At least, that is the premise of this well documented book. The book was written in and about South Africa with 11 official languages, but the insights and findings go far beyond any particular geographic setting in their profound implications for democratizing psychology on a global scale. Strous documents in detail the connections between psychology and the apartheid-style psychology imposed on the portion of South Africa's population who were Black or Colored. South Africa provides a prime example of why multicultural competency is essential in any society.

All societies are multicultural with the uneven distribution of power across defined groups within those societies. All societies are experiencing rapid social change and transition to meet the needs and demands of culturally defined groups within each society. This transition from discrimination toward cultural sensitivity has profound implications for the field of psychology. Strous is careful to document how profoundly apartheid shaped the theory and practice of psychology in South Africa, where "multicultural" differences in society were actually used to defend discrimination in favor of Whites even though South Africa's 77 percent Black population represents an overwhelming numerical majority. The consequences of White superiority were clearly destructive to all sectors of South African society and these "mistakes" are documented in detail.

Strous advocates a "balanced" alternative to the practice of applied psychology and therapy. This balance acknowledges the mistakes and builds toward positive alternatives much as the policy of "reconciliation" in South Africa has rejected the goals of revenge and advocated a more positive alternative. Issues of Human Rights and the democratization of psychology takes a post-modern constructivist perspective toward the practice of psychology that highlights the importance of multicultural competencies and training mental health care providers to be more sensitive to both cultural similarities and differences.

Strous's own research on the training of therapists was based on the Triad Training Model where a counselor, coached-client, pro-counselor and anticounselor interact in a role played interview to articulate the positive and negative internal dialogue of the counselor and coached-client. We can only learn from our mistakes if we know that we have just made a mistake. The balance of immediate and continuous positive and negative feedback from a pro and anti perspective guides the therapist toward increased awareness and sensitivity to implicit bias and covert racism in therapy. The pro and anti perspectives provide a balance in training the therapists to their own implicit "anticlient" and "pro-client" assumptions in Strous's own unique adaptation of the Triad Training Model.

This book appears in the "Contributions in Psychology" series as one more example of how the field of applied psychology meets the needs of our rapidly changing society. Each book in this series has advanced our understanding of how psychology contributes to civilization, one small step at a time. While we know a great deal about the world around us, we know relatively little about our inner psychological world, how it functions, how it is changed, and how it facilitates the change process. Strous goes a long ways toward helping us better understand ourselves as multicultural persons living in multicultural societies. This book provides a valuable lesson for those who question the importance of multicultural competencies in the field of psychology.

Paul Pedersen
University of Hawaii
March 4, 2003

Preface

South Africa's transition from a racially discriminatory state to a "rainbow nation" valuing human diversity and equality has required vast shifts in social ideology. South Africa is a country that has undergone far-reaching change, accompanied, at least in theory and design, with the replacement of formalized discrimination. Mirroring these processes of transformation, there has been and continues to be a need to substitute discriminatory mental health practices, previously accepted as conventional, with more culturally and racially sensitive alternatives.

Throughout the world, contextually inappropriate psychological models are frequently imposed on members of nondominant groups, leading to oppression in the field of mental health. This book focuses on how practices of mental health and racism have played out in the South African scenario and how they reflect assumptions concerning "White superiority" and "Black inferiority." These practices and assumptions are then juxtaposed against competing ideals of the human rights movement, the democratization of psychotherapy, and the ethos of postmodernism and social constructionism.

The book indicates a need for flexibility in mental health provision beyond automatic adherence to Eurocentric or idealized American norms. South Africa is a multicultural country with 11 official languages reflecting its diversity. The current population is approximately 43 million, of which about 77 percent have been identified as "Black," 9 percent "Colored," 2.5 percent "Asian," and 10.5 percent "White" (Statistics for South Africa, 2000. Cited in Sturgeon, 2002). South African psychology is faced with the need to transcend its historical over reliance on European and American theorizing that frequently dominate despite the diverse needs of a multicultural population. Psychology as practiced under the apartheid regime had potential to undermine clients from subordinate groups.

Counselors from South Africa and other countries can learn much from each other, in terms of both their mistakes as well as their successes. Issues confronting South African counselors are in some ways unique, but they also resonate with international literature and experiences. The book acknowledges cultural sensitivity in counseling as a global human rights issue. Psychotherapists who operate in multicultural and multiracial settings are often unconscious of their own ideological biases, while racial and cultural sensitivity training programs are limited. The heterogeneous needs of diverse groups require mental health practitioners to carefully reflect upon the appropriateness of their assumptions and practices. A failure by practitioners to develop cultural competency and to deliver nondiscriminatory services would perpetuate broader social inequities within the practice of psychology, counseling, and mental health service delivery.

The book is divided into three sections. Part I, "Apartheid-Style Psychology," illustrates how professional training for mental health practitioners is generally inadequate on matters pertaining to race and racism and how therapists may be influenced by prevailing racist ideologies, unaware of how their racial and cultural prejudices translate into discriminatory work practices and ignorant of the power of their own elite discourses. Part II, "Alternatives to Apartheid-Style Psychology," investigates positions related to racial and cultural sensitivity that stand in contradiction to the negative and disruptive positions identified in Part I. Part III, "Training Models," describes the Triad Model and proposes a new multicultural and multiracial sensitivity training model for further research. The Afterword summarizes some of the main points of the book and suggests areas for future research.

I would like to acknowledge Gill Eagle and Gill Straker from the University of the Witwatersrand, Johannesburg and Paul Pedersen from the University of Alabama at Birmingham who were influential in helping me to arrive at the ideas contained in this book. I am also deeply indebted to my wife, children and parents for their support during the writing of the book. Finally, to the reader of this book, I express my appreciation and hope that you will use its content to further develop equitable services for those in need.

Part I

Apartheid-Style Psychology

This section illustrates how professional training for mental health practitioners is generally inadequate on matters pertaining to race and racism and how therapists, unaware that racial prejudices translate into discriminatory work practices and ignorant of the power of their own elite discourses, may be influenced by prevailing racist ideologies. Chapter 1 focuses on the manner in which practices of mental health and racism have played out in the South African scenario and reflect assumptions concerning "White superiority." The ideological landscape on which apartheid was predicated, the institutionalization of racism via apartheid legislation, and the social consequences which ensued with particular reference to group consciousness are discussed. More specifically, an enduring impact of apartheid ideology on South African psychologists is suggested. In Chapter 2, the role of mental health services in replicating and perpetuating discrimination is investigated. Institutions that provided separate and unequal treatment for Blacks and Whites, intentional prejudice amongst some South African psychologists, inadvertent collusion with the status quo through uncritical research, and shortages of personnel that resulted and continue to result in inferior mental health services for the majority of the population are explored. Chapter 3 describes how counselor encapsulation can lead to misdiagnoses, distorted or inadequate knowledge of diverse client worldviews, and the rendering of inappropriate mental health services.

Mental Health and Racism

INTRODUCTION

The theory and practice of psychotherapy in any context is influenced by its host culture (Richards, 1997). According to Richards (1997), psychologists who are members of cultural and psychological communities necessarily share those communities' psychological character in some degree. A critical, reflexive analysis as to how psychotherapy and psychological theory have developed within particular social and political contexts is imperative if therapists socialized within racist societies and exposed to racism within their discipline are to achieve self-awareness. Even the most self-consciously "antiracist" people may appear retrospectively racist from a critically reflective position (Richards, 1997, xiv).

THE EARLY COLONIAL ERA

Deficit models of Black inferiority and assumptions of White superiority have been advanced and perpetuated by mental health professionals, sometimes overtly and sometimes unintentionally, since at least the colonial era. The predominant view of Africans held by colonialists in both Europe and South Africa was that of inferior beings (Foster, 1993).

Colonialists initially conceived of Blacks as exempt from madness, which afflicted some Europeans. Blacks were considered "primitives" whose undeveloped civilizations did not impose on them responsibilities required of "tragic" European man. Rousseau (1762), in his *Social Contract and Discourses*, conceived of the Black as a "noble savage" who led the joyful, light-hearted existence of a brute with no fixed abode or articulate speech, and whose needs were easily satisfied. Because Blacks operated in a natural state of impulse-driven instinctiveness, reasoned colonialists, it followed that they would not have to endure mental illness, which was linked to being civilized (Littlewood & Lipsedge, 1997). Many social scientists have since concluded that people of color are mentally unsophisticated and incapable of mental disorders (Carter, 1995, p. 32).

The early colonial perspective, that freedom from civilizing restraints allowed Blacks to remain happy, provided an expedient rationale for advocating not overloading the lucky native with responsibility (Littlewood & Lipsedge, 1997, p. 34). Behind most racial discrimination is the idea that members of one racial group, because of their supposed superior endowment and greater innate ability, are cause of their supposed superior endowment and greater innate ability, are entitled to privileges not accorded to members of another group (Tobias, 1972, p. 7). The frequent inferiority of mental health services that is provided to Black patients and the frequent underrepresentation of Black mental health practitioners reflect the enduring impact of early colonial prejudices, which held that mental health facilities should be reserved for "sophisticated" Whites.

The idea that "primitives" could not become mentally ill quickly evolved during the colonial era into the idea that in some sense they already were ill. Littlewood and Lipsedge (1997) summarize this perspective:

The African was simultaneously "a child, an idiot and a madman" (Jordan, 1968), Kipling's "half devil-half child." Primitive religion was "organized schizophrenia," magic the "pathology of culture," the savage an "obsessional neurotic." Native healers were epileptics, hysterics or neurotics. The mentally ill shared the primitiveness of tribal men.... If the insane regressed to a primitive state of mind because of the stresses of society, the Blacks were already there. Among them madness was, as it were, spread out thin—their normal condition. (p. 35)

The notion that Blacks were not exempt from mental illness but were habitually crazed surfaced and gained credibility in the nineteenth century. Intolerance and patronizing attitudes toward Blacks and indigenous healing still endure today, partly as a legacy of early colonial ideologies.

SCIENTIFIC RACISM

With the emancipation of slaves in the nineteenth century, which potentially allowed Blacks access to European civilization, cultural hypotheses for subjugating the "noble savage," which characterized early colonialism, were no longer sufficient to justify racial discrimination, because freed slaves could hypothetically be socialized into mainstream society. Justifications for oppression now became couched in popular genetic explanations of the day, which embraced the idea that Blacks could not change their constitutional inferiority (Littlewood & Lipsedge, 1997).

The natural sciences were held in high esteem in the nineteenth century and a proliferation of biological theories endorsed the notion of Black inferiority. Science "proved" that Whites possessed willpower, self-control and reason and that Blacks loved "melody and ostentation" but lacked judgment. Blacks' brains were suggested to be smaller than Whites' brains and their genitals were suggested to be larger than those of Whites, reflecting sexual extremes belonging to an age of awakening consciousness or nascent intelligence (Bevis, 1921; Jung, 1930; Lind, 1913; Littlewood & Lipsedge, 1997; O'Malley, 1914; Thomas & Sillen, 1972).

In the 1920s, psychologists such as Yerkes, Goddard, Terman, and Brigham concluded that races differed in intelligence. These psychologists participated in eugenic practices that contributed to the restriction of immigrants to the United States (Kamin, 1974). The eugenics movement, led by Jensen, provided a highly quotable string of rationalizations for the resurgence of racism in America and Britain (Heather, 1976, p. 126). In South Africa, M.L. Fick and J.A.J. van Rensburg came to hold similar views in the 1930s (Foster, 1993).

Genetic deficit hypotheses postulated that minority groups in Britain and America were deficient in desirable genes and that this impacted adversely on either their personality or intelligence (Jensen, 1969; Rushton, 1988; Shockley, 1971; Shuey,

1966). Hernstein (1994), following a genetic deficit line, has claimed that permanent genetic differences account for high and low levels of achievement, and that affirmative remedial programs cannot bridge the genetic gap between racial groups.

A clear error in arguments advocating a race, intelligence, and genetics link is the disregard of how intelligence is measured, and whether intelligence tests and other achievement tests are valid and reliable in different social contexts. Hendersen (1976) and Heather (1976) view intelligence testing as providing a standard whereby the continued meritocratic distribution of opportunities based on White middle-class norms is perpetuated. Intelligence testing is based on a conformity model, which assumes the normal distribution of characteristics and behaviors throughout a population. The graph of the normal distribution is a smooth, bell-shaped curve, indicating a concentration of high frequencies in the center of the distribution (the average range of intellectual functioning) and increasingly lower frequencies toward either tail (higher or lower ranges of intellectual functioning). The importance of the standard normal distribution is that it permits the determination of percentile ranks or points, which helps to locate an individual within a distribution (McKall, 1986). The major racial implication of the conformity model in the United States has been the imposition of majority norms on minority clients (Ridley, 1995). An individual's or group's relative standing may be grossly misrepresented as deficient through lack of comparability of test norms (Anastasi, 1976, pp. 88–96). Counselors who generalize culturally universal, or etic, norms and techniques across cultures, violate the principle of norm-referenced interpretation because an individual should only be compared with a group of people who have matching characteristics (Ridley, 1995, pp. 49–50).

THE CULTURAL DEFICIT MODEL

Nazi Germany applied the scientific method with fervor to the issue of race. Because of Nazi atrocities perpetrated in the service of racial "cleansing," racio-genetic explanations became unpopular and were vigorously refuted. Discrimination based on "genetic inferiority" came to be considered pathological itself. In opposition to scientific racism, the cultural deficit model asserted that, under the yoke of oppression in Britain and America, minority cultures had been compromised and were socially rather than biologically disadvantaged. Cultural background, it was contended, resulted in minorities being unable to compete with dominant groups in society.

Cultural deficit models, which were developed to counter genetic deficiency theories, may unintentionally perpetuate racism by implying that racial ethnic groups do not possess "the right culture" (Atkinson, Morten, & Sue, 1993). Racism can profoundly compromise the lives and psychological integrity of its victims (Carter, 1994; Jones, 1992; Landrine & Klonoff, 1996; Vera & Feagin, 1995). However, the implication that the African American is invariably and necessarily compromised by cultural deficit has presented difficulties (Richards, 1997, pp. 241–242). Implicit in the concept of "cultural deprivation" has been the assumption that the standards of the dominant White middle class represent norms by which all other cultures can be measured (Thomas & Sillen, 1972, p. 68).

Cultural deprivation studies usefully highlight obstacles facing Blacks, but often assume that Blacks are *inevitably* damaged by their surroundings (Carter, 1995; Owusu-Bempah & Howitt, 1999). There is a tendency by White psychologists upholding Euro-American philosophy to ignore contrasting research and demonstrable behaviors of Blacks attesting to their strengths and abilities (Carter, 1995; Johnson & Wilderson, 1969; Mays, 1985; Thomas & Sillen, 1972).

A consequence of being referred to as "deficient" may be the setting of exaggerated goals for those so labeled to prove themselves; or its opposite, sparing them the stresses of responsibility. Either way, Blacks may be excluded from opportunities afforded to Whites. In the field of mental health, opportunities for Black professionals and treatment for Black patients have been inferior to those for Whites.

Whether Black "deficiency" is located in biological or cultural arguments is irrelevant if, in the final analysis, the problem remains "at the level of the Black individual or family and does not begin to deal with forces in the larger society responsible for creating these conditions" (Barnes, 1980, p. 110). There is a need to acknowledge ideological factors that operate in the social construction of race.

THE SOCIAL CONSTRUCTION OF RACE

Racially discriminatory practices frequently assume that:

1.   Races are pure and distinct entities;
2.   All members of a race look, think, and behave alike; and
3.   Some races are better than others, with some falling "right outside the magic circle of love and brotherhood" because they are inferior (Tobias, 1972, p. 36).

The concept of race owes its popularity to a variety of ideological and cultural factors (Richards, 1997, p. x). As a pseudoscientific construct that attributes psychological characteristics to members of groups, race may be regarded as a fiction (Carter, 1995, p. 15; Helmes, 1990, p. 4; Pedersen, 1988, p. viii; Ponterrotto & Pedersen, 1993, p. 6). The political importance of racial identities has been increasingly emphasized and race as a biological concept has become increasingly controversial (Yee, Fairchild, Weizmann, & Wyatt, 1993). Race as a social scientific construct refers "to group characteristics that in popular ideology [not fact] are carried in the blood (i.e., skin-color)" (Johnson, 1990, p. 41).

Carter (1995, p. 15) views race as a socio-political designation that one individual uses to assign worth to another individual or group based on racial group membership (pp. 15, 225). This is in line with Social Identity Theory, which explains in-group favoritism and out-group discrimination on the understanding that, in order to boost self-esteem, individuals try to view the social category with which the self is identified as positively as possible in comparison to other social groups (Tajfel, 1978). Social Identity Theory recognizes the process whereby similarities within "racialized" groups and differences between groups are exaggerated or accentuated.

Race group membership fundamentally affects self-definition and affects intrapersonal, interpersonal, and intergroup processes (Korf & Schoeman, 1996, p. 213). The view that race is socially constructed—an empty signifier with no ontological validity—permits its analysis in terms of relationships of dominance (Carrim, 2000; Miles, 1989). However, the social construction of race is not fully appreciated in psychiatric circles (Fernando, 1988, 1991).

RACISM AND WHITE IDENTITY

A number of writers (e.g., Carter & Helms, 1990; Katz, 1982; Patel et al., 2000; Stern, 1987; Trepagnier, 1994; Wong, 1994) have recently taken issue with the focus in psychology and the social sciences on race and racism as it affects Blacks. For these writers, the emphasis on what it is to be "Black" detracts from a need to scrutinize the meaning of "Whiteness."

Little has been published on racism as it affects Whites (Katz, 1982, p. 7). The assumption that race is associated only with Blacks and that racism is harmful only to the oppressed provides no information about how Whites feel about themselves as members of a racial group, and the harmful effects of racism on Whites (Helms, 1984; Carter, 1995). For Katz (1982), the focus on Blacks as victims targets the symptoms of racism, rather than the victimizer who is the cause. Katz cites a number of writers who suggest that racism could be dehumanizing for Whites as well as for Blacks, and that the lack of insight on the part of many Whites that there are alternative worldviews different to dominant White norms suggests a lack of insight as to self-identity (e.g., Allen, 1971; Beck, 1973; Bidol, 1971; Citron, 1969; Cobbs, 1972; Du Bois, 1903; Kovel, 1970). Katz (1982) is of the opinion that "racism has severely hindered White people's psychological and intellectual development. In psychological terms racism has deluded Whites into a false sense of superiority.... In intellectual terms racism has resulted in miseducation about the realities of history, the contributions of Third World people, and the role of White people in present-day culture" (p. 15).

Overfocusing on the adverse psychological effects that racism has for Whites in terms of its dehumanizing consequences could reinforce the central racist narrative that the experiences of White people are more important than those of Blacks (Hooks, 1996). Nevertheless, in order to function appropriately and sensitively in rapidly changing multicultural/racial societies, human service professionals must be aware of their own life experiences and how these have contributed to the development of their prejudices (Sturgeon, 2002).

A recent call has been for Whites to "do race;" that is, to critically interrogate their own privileges afforded to them by their race (Wong, 1994). "We read about White researchers' forays into "urban ghettos" to study, research and ameliorate the plight and conditions of the "colored" poor without reflecting and problematizing *their* race and class," states Wong (1994, p. 135). According to Macleod and Durrheim (in press), "Black" has been exoticized, rendered strange, and opened to audible and visible scrutiny, while "Whiteness" remains tacit and hidden, a normalized absent trace. Casting Blacks as Other represents a pathologized presence that relies on the normalized absent trace of Whiteness for definition (Derrida, 1978,1983; Phoenix and Woollett, 1991, cited in Macleod and Durrheim, in press). What remains hidden is the bias of those doing the defining (Macleod and Durrheim, in press).

Frankenberg (1993, cited in Patel et al., 2000) states that "Whiteness, as a set of normative cultural practices is visible most clearly to those it definitively excludes and those to whom it does violence. Those who are securely housed within its borders usually do not examine it" (p. 228).

Taking cognizance of the issue of White racial identity, Helms and Pipers' (1994) revised developmental theory of White racial identity levels proposes a six-status process:

1. Contact,
2. Disintegration,
3. Reintegration,
4. Pseudo-independence,
5. Immersion–Emersion, and
6. Autonomy.

These statuses are divided into two phases:

1. The abandonment of a racist identity (Contact–Reintegration); and
2. The establishment of a nonracial White identity (Immersion–Autonomy).

Carter (1995) advocates that Whites must accept their Whiteness, understand the cultural meanings of being White, and develop a self-concept devoid of any element associated with racial superiority. However, few strategies or materials have been designed to raise the consciousness of White people, to help them identify racism in themselves and others, and to develop skills to facilitate change in the White community (Katz, 1982). Multicultural education programs, aimed at breaking down cultural barriers, tend to emphasize appreciation of cultural differences without sufficiently scrutinizing the issue of White racism (Katz, 1982). White counselor self-awareness of racial identity is an important variable that is required for developing multicultural competence (Richardson & Molinaro, 1996).

Katz (1982) points out that some White-on-White training groups have been developed by Whites to explore their racism (e.g., Cleaver, 1968; Moore, 1973; Terry, 1970). Stern (1987) has used terms from transactional analysis to try uncovering possible hidden racism of White counselors in the Netherlands at the individual and institutional levels. These endeavors are compatible with calls for Whites to try breaking down prejudice and discrimination within their own communities (Bennett, 1966; Coppard & Steinwachs, 1970; Edler, 1974; Knowles & Prewitt, 1969; Welsing, 1974).

In the field of psychiatry, Fernando (1989) contends that only once a psychiatrist appreciates the social nature of racism, and psychiatry's involvement in racism, will that psychiatrist be ready to grapple with cultural aspects of an encounter: "The promotion of cultural sensitivity without challenging racism may result in the reinforcement of racism by masking it and thereby inducing complacency" (Fernando, 1989, p. 167).

Patel et al. (2000) state that "we need to recognize our relative freedom from injustice, not to engender guilt, but to enable us to be open, to give up "being special" and to start to talk to each other about our part in redressing the imbalance of hurt and injustice" (p. 11). The Anticlient–Proclient Model proposed in Chapter 6 of this book represents an attempt to facilitate self-reflection on issues pertaining to White counselor identity, with specific reference to counselors who were socialized within apartheid South Africa.

APARTHEID

The idea of race has held a tenacious grip on the minds of South Africans (Tobias, 1972). Racism operated in South Africa from the arrival of the first White settlers in various ideological and institutional forms (Foster & Louw Potgieter, 1992,

p. 336). Scientific racism and cultural deficit understandings were accorded different significance at different points in time, but both pointed to the "inferiority" of Black psychological functioning in order to justify White dominance. Domination of South Africa's indigenous peoples by Whites was justified with reference to racist European ideologies.

The division of Whites and nonWhites in every sphere of South African life was ruthlessly enforced under apartheid. "Race became a national neurosis of the obsessional variety" (Tobias, 1972, p. 1), with every aspect of society based on differential treatment of the races.

Structures of White domination were entrenched under the apartheid system via "separate development" legislation. The policy of separate development aimed to protect White "nationhood," through the splitting up of Whites, Colored, Indians and "Bantu nations." Dr. D.F. Malan declared that only by the policy of apartheid could the White race be saved from African domination, and he won the 1948 General Election on the premise that conflict and prejudice would disappear if extensive contact between groups were eliminated.

The apartheid regime enjoyed ardent support from Afrikaner nationalists. Drawing from Calvinist theological dichotomies between the "elected" and the "damned," Afrikaner national ideology had defined Afrikaners as a chosen people on a divine mission for their own land and nation, and rejected any form of leveling between Blacks and Whites. Afrikaner nationalism thus constituted a powerful ideological device for the creation of social identities and racial group consciousness in South Africa (Foster and Louw-Potgieter, 1992, p. 369). Racial attitudes and Calvinist theology were intertwined in a manner that facilitated Afrikaner group cohesiveness and Black subordination (Du Toit, 1983; Foster & Louw-Potgieter, 1992; MacCrone, 1937).

The defining variable of apartheid ideology was "difference." With the demise of the Nazi regime and its vulgar racism based on the superiority and inferiority of racial groups, it was more acceptable in political circles to refer to cultural differences between people than to White supremacy (Magubane, 1979). Defined and imposed by the state, "difference" provided the rationale for creating a mosaic of racially and ethnically defined political and geographical entities (Nkomo, Mkwanazi-Twala & Carrim, 1995).

Racial Segregation

The view that Blacks were culturally different culminated in their alienation from White society through the "Bantustan" or homelands policy. The rationale of this policy was to provide separate territories for each of the "nations" that inhabited South Africa, and resulted in the forced mass removal of approximately 3.5 million, mostly Black people, from their places of abode (Platzky & Walker, 1985).

Massive social engineering resulted in the splitting of Black families, poverty, and oppression (Duncan & Rock, 1995; Richter, 1994). Legislative enactments swept away common law safeguards of human rights, while the system of parliamentary supremacy disallowed the courts from challenging oppressive state legislation (Carpenter, 1987; Sachs, 1985; van der Vyfer, 1985). The constitutional system of partial democracy allowed the government to ride roughshod over human rights safeguards in the common law without alienating the minority White electorate.

The apartheid system strongly affected group identities by encouraging the perception that South Africans could be neatly categorized into discrete racial groups and geographical locations. Race played a major part in determining a person's legal status and a plethora of legislation aimed at population control was spawned. The Populations Registration Act of 1950 provided for the registration of the population and the issuing of identity cards. In terms of the Prohibition of Mixed Marriages Act of 1949, marriages between Whites and nonWhites were void and of no effect. Section 16 of the Immorality Act of 1957 prohibited sexual relationships between Whites and nonWhites. The Group Areas Act reserved certain areas for the ownership and occupation of persons of a certain race. The sale and letting of such land to persons of other races was restricted.

Three main levels of segregation in South African society could be distinguished under apartheid:

1.   The segregation of public places such as washrooms, waiting rooms, railway carriages, and other public areas (microsegregation).
2.   The segregation of Whites and nonWhites in terms of the neighborhoods in which they lived in urban areas (mezzosegregation).
3.   The segregation of whole peoples in distinct territories set up as *native reserves* (macrosegregation) (van den Berghe, 1970, cited in Giddens, 1989, p. 258).

Inequality of Services and Opportunities

Legislation controlling the movement of Blacks established personal and interpersonal attitudes of racial difference and exclusivity, based on the assumption that Blacks were inferior and entitled to fewer resources and privileges (Nkomo et al., 1995, p. 265). Inferior public amenities, education, occupational opportunities, and health facilities were provided for Blacks, and indicated the inferior status assigned to them.

The Reservation of Separate Amenities Act of 1953 provided for the reservation of separate public facilities, premises, or vehicles, or portions thereof, for the exclusive use of different races. The facilities did not have to be equal or even available at all for members of a particular racial group, and were frequently inferior or lacking for Blacks.

The educational system was also legally segregated along racial lines. Financial allocations to the educational needs of each racial group were grossly disparate in favor of White education (Cooper, Nicholas, Seedat, & Statmann, 1990; Duncan & Rock, 1995). Facilities in African schools were inadequate, and Black students perceived themselves as being trained in apartheid schools for low paying jobs and subordinate social positions (Nkomo et al., 1995, pp. 270–271). Blacks could not attend White universities without special ministerial permission.

In South African schools, textbooks, a likely influence in processes of political socialization and racist ideology development (Foster, 1986), covered the history of White groups at the expense of Blacks (Auerbach, 1965; Dean, Hartmann, & Katzen, 1983), and repeatedly intimated at White superiority and Black inferiority (Du Preez, 1983). White schools were required to include in their curricula a paramilitary component, a primary aim being to ensure unquestioning conformity to, and support for, the apartheid system (Cooper, et al., 1990). Guidance programs at Black schools aimed to inculcate values of conformity and acquiescence, and could be described as "curricula for servitude and docility" (Cooper et al., 1990, p. 10). Apartheid education fuelled bloated ethnocentricity and impeded society's capacity to conceive of different social relations (Hickson & Kriegler, 1996, p. 61).

The Job Reservation Act, the Native Building Workers Act and the Industrial Conciliation Act protected White workers from displacement by Black workers. These laws were modified after 1978, but for over twenty years the execution of their provisions perpetuated racism in promoting White supremacy and in ensuring the placement of Blacks in inferior unskilled and semi-skilled occupational positions (Nkomo et al., 1995, p. 264).

Enormous disparities of wealth and opportunity, together with sharp contrasts enshrined in law, have therefore divided White and so-called "nonWhite South Africans" (Giddens, 1990). White South Africans belong to an economically privileged group. Many Whites have seen in the historical nexus of class and color proof that Blacks are bio-genetically predestined to lower class positions, when in fact White dominance of central power institutions has determined the distribution of opportunities (Rhoodie, 1983, pp. 478–480). As elsewhere, race and class have frequently cohered in South Africa as testimony to the effects of racist policies and practices.

From early childhood, race meant privilege and power or the lack of it (Dawes, 1985). The inferior position of the Black nanny or domestic worker attests to this. The majority of White children were raised in homes where domestic workers were denied the right to emotional reciprocity and mutual relationship obligations (Straker, 1989; Wulfsohn, 1988). In 1984, approximately 76 percent of White families had at least one domestic worker (Goodwin, 1984), almost without exception Black or so-called "Colored." The domestic worker has often been reduced to a labor unit rather than thought of as a person (Cock, 1980; Mohutsioa-Makhudu, 1989; Preston-Whyte, 1976). Until the late 1990s, the conditions of work of domestic workers were inadequately protected in law. Domestic workers, usually women unless gardeners, have been an ultra-exploited group in South Africa (Hickson & Strous, 1993).

The inferior status assigned to Blacks is further reflected in the fact that English and Afrikaans, a language largely derived from Dutch, were assigned as the official languages in South Africa up until the post-apartheid era. Fewer than half a percent of Black South Africans do not speak a traditional language (Rhoodie, 1983), but Blacks have been expected to communicate to their White compatriots in English or Afrikaans. The divide and rule strategy of the apartheid regime was to contend that Black South Africans did not form one homogenous group, but a number of heterogeneous groups with their own discernible languages to be spoken in circumscribed geographical areas (Finchelescu & Nyawose, 1998). Black South Africans have queried why Whites find difficulty in learning African languages when they have had to learn English or Afrikaans (Swartz, Drennan & Crawford, 1997). It is a feature of racism that speakers of "refined" European languages have been virtuously represented as rational, moral, civilized and capable of abstract thinking, while "inferior" civilizations have been supposedly marked by linguistic incapacity and inability to assimilate (Goldberg, 1994, p. 71). In an inversion of power relations (Maakhe, 1994), the majority population had their languages accorded secondary status to languages originating in Western Europe.

The Impact of Apartheid Socialization on White Psychologists

South Africa's first democratic election was held in April 1994. Archbishop Desmond Tutu, the Nobel Peace Prize winner, compared South Africa's political transition to a rainbow over the social battlefield, symbolizing unity in a multi-colored diversity and a sacred covenant binding South Africans in harmony. As remarkable a transition as South Africa has undergone, it has, however, inherited the social devastation wreaked by the apartheid years. Rainbows are up in the sky, states Schlemmer (1996); closer to the ground, racial feelings threaten the potential good-will of the new order. Notions of "Mandela magic" and the "rainbow nation" are wonderful, unifying symbols, but they may conceal a lack of attention to the serious problem of race, racism and racial identity (Gobodo-Madikizela, 1997).

In the view of Bhekhi Peterson (1999):

South Africa, despite its democratically elected government, is still very much a society that is "structured in racial dominance." Political reforms have not been matched by achievements or equalities in the economic, social, educational and cultural spheres. As Mbeki keeps on reminding everyone: South Africa is one country with two nations: one rich and white and one poor and black. Given the continuing verity that many social experiences "are not simply 'colored' by race" but "work through race," it follows that "race is the modality through which class is lived," the form in which it is appropriated and "fought through." As a result, the stark inequalities in wealth, education and social amenities assume a pronounced racial character. …The ideas of racial superiority and inferiority, in as much as they have been contested throughout this century, continue to inform political cultures and identities in South Africa, in both crass and subtle ways. (pp. 9–10)

Private preferences have led to informal racial segregation in post apartheid South Africa, (Goldberg, 1994). Racial schisms and racist attitudes have not been swept away by the repeal of enactments that legitimated them. As elsewhere, in South Africa ambivalent racial attitudes may be characterized by superficial tolerance superimposed upon underlying covert negative emotion. White liberal attitudes may coexist with strict social distance from Blacks and subtle racism (Crosby, Bromley & Saxe, 1980; Duckitt, 1992; Durrheim, 2000; Kinder & Sears, 1981; Kinder, 1986; Lea, 1996; McConahay, 1986; Preston-Whyte, 1976).

Major themes pervading notions of modern "racism" (e.g., Gaertner & Dovidio, 1986; McConahay, 1986) are that overt acts of racism, which are intentional and relatively easy to detect, may be on the decline, whereas covert racism, which is subtle and often beyond conscious awareness, may be increasing. Unlike intentional overt or intentional covert racism, which involve malicious intent, unintentional covert racism involves nonmaleficence (Ridley, 1995). Overt racism is unlikely to be challenged and is treacherous because of a lack of knowledge of wrongdoing on the part of its inadvertent perpetrators (Pedersen, 1997; Ponterotto & Pedersen, 1993). An observation by Ridley (1995) that "counselors, in many ways, are socialized and trained to behave as racists without even knowing it" (p. 39) is compatible with understandings of modern racism, which describe how persons who regard themselves as nonprejudiced and nondiscriminating can espouse egalitarian values, sympathies with victims of injustice, promote policies of racial equality, and yet behave in racist ways (Ponterotto & Pedersen, 1993).

Despite psychology's standing as a liberal humanity, South African psychologists, socialized in a cultural milieu that encouraged racial separation and that condoned racial inequality, may, even in the postapartheid era be influenced, inadvertently, by their apartheid socialization. As Nkomo et al. (1995) have stated:

Apartheid explicitly fragmented the socio-economic and political landscape of South Africa along racial lines. The theological and quasi-scientific justifications provided the raison d'être for the constitutional entrenchment of racism and the proliferation of racist laws. It ideologically affected the consciousness of South Africans and cast them in racial moulds. It also ensured that legally defined racial groups lived different, unequal and separate lives. (pp. 265–266)

According to the social contact hypothesis, a lack of contact between members of various groups may lead to prejudice and outgroup discrimination (Ashmore, 1970). Contact in situations that enhance awareness of group identification and fortify boundaries between groups may strengthen group identity fixation (Bornman & Appelgryn, 1999). The apartheid regime focused obsessively on pigeonholing groups as a means of maintaining power, and emphasized group differences rather than common humanity (Sifrin, Friedman, & Bellar, 1997). As a result, groups acquired a siege mentality toward each other and people perceived others through the filter of group stereotypes rather than through open and healthy personal experiences (Sifrin, Friedman, & Bellar, 1997). It would have been impossible for South African therapists not to experience the pull of social and racial identity, and it would be difficult for them to magically overcome biases with the ushering in of a new government.

Therapist socialization in a racist and ethnocentric society may compromise effective multicultural and interracial counseling (Bloombaum, Yamamoto, & James, 1968; Casas, 1984; Vontress, 1981). Even in the context of American democracy, it has been noted that, "it may be difficult for persons removed from the ghetto to accept the style of life of those who are part of it and to refrain from attempting to impose a Puritan-ethic-tinged morality upon it" (Sager, Brayboy, & Waxenburg cited by Jones & Seagull, 1977, p. 852).

In an exercise conducted at the University of Cape Town (Sturgeon, 2002), students in the Department of Social Development were asked to write an "Ethnic Autobiography," tracing their life history in terms of their own and other ethnic groups, how this awareness was developed, and their current attitudes. The responses of the White students indicated immense guilt and anger concerning their ignorance of the effects of apartheid, and shock at their own acceptance of the stereotypes of Black people. The effectiveness of the apartheid system in separating people and the strength of its propaganda became apparent, indicating the need for multicultural self-awareness on the part of helping professionals.

In the view of Cooper et al., (1990), psychology as a discipline, a body of knowledge, and as a profession, has been compatible with a system of social control based on racism, coercion, and brutality. These authors contend that organized psychology in South Africa generally accommodated, contributed to, and failed to oppose the development of the apartheid state.

White South African counselors subjected to processes of apartheid ideology would have access to a range of competing psychological literature and experiences, encouraging and instructing them in effective interpersonal relating. However, the legacy of what was enforced, and what frequently remains, de facto segregation of Whites and Blacks, may continue to adversely affect White counselor–Black client dyadic processes.

SUMMARY

In South Africa, racist ideologies found expression in proclaimed state policies of racial differentiation and separation. Under apartheid, rights and privileges were extended to the White minority at the expense of gross violations to the rights of the unenfranchized majority. Apartheid ideology and a pathological social political structure resulted in frustrated aspirations, widespread poverty and suffering for millions of Blacks.

The apartheid attempt to crystallize ethnic consciousness (Dawes, 1986) encouraged the perception that South Africans could be neatly categorized into discrete racial groups and separated from one another. The pernicious and enthusiastic execution of apartheid law provisions ensured that South Africans led racially segregated, divided, and unequal lives. Thus, White South African psychologists working interracially may be hindered by sentiments reflective of conservative psychological research and practice, racist ideologies rooted in colonialism, scientific racism, and notions of cultural deficit. White psychologists who were largely removed from the psychosocial experiences that affect many of their potential clients as a result of apartheid segregation and socialization policies, may also experience anxiety in interracial counseling contexts; aware that they hold truncated understandings of Black worldviews.

South African psychologists have been exposed to not only the socializing influences of Grand Apartheid, but also to a profession which in many instances replicated racial discrimination, and, in violation of basic human rights, perpetuated social injustice. This will be elaborated upon in Chapter 2, where our discussion turns to mental health services in South Africa that have frequently failed its majority Black population.

2

Mental Health Services in South Africa: Separate and Unequal

INSTITUTIONAL CARE

South Africa's history of racial separation and inequality found expression in its mental health institutions. Racial segregation of mental asylums in South Africa, from the 1800s to 1990, facilitated racialized diagnostic and treatment practices between "European" and "Native" patient populations (Foster, 1993; S. Swartz, 1995a). The Robben Island asylum, opened in 1847, was formally segregated by 1890. This was a time when social Darwinism was influential, reflected in the words of the Superintendent of Robben Island who stated that: "No comparison can in fairness be instituted between the lunacy of savages and uneducated natives and the derangements of nervous systems met with among highly organized individuals living at the headlong pace of the 19th Century" (de Villiers, 1971, cited by Foster, 1993, p. 204).

In the 1970s, both the American Psychiatric Association (APA) and the World Health Organization (WHO) voiced concern that Blacks were receiving inferior treatment in South African psychiatric institutions. Both the APA and the WHO reports focused primarily on inadequate services at government funded psychiatric facilities at the privately owned Smith-Mitchell and Company institutions. The Smith-Mitchell facilities under contract to the South African government provided racially segregated care on a per diem basis for involuntary psychiatric patients referred from state institutions.

The APA report (1979) found disparate amounts being spent on mental health care for White patients and for Black patients. The psychiatric care provided at the Smith-Mitchell institutions for Black patients was inadequate; the psychiatrists could speak none of the Black languages; facilities for patients were converted mine compounds with insufficient ventilation; toilet facilities were inadequate and dining facilities overcrowded; and the number of beds provided were insufficient. The Department of Health had informed officials of the APA that there was a shortage of beds because Blacks prefer to sleep on the floor. The Department also argued that patients without shoes preferred to go barefoot. Patients interviewed reported having been beaten or assaulted by staff or having witnessed other patients being assaulted. The staff was grossly inadequate in number to provide decent rehabilitative treatment and nurses were under-trained. There were a high number of needless deaths among patients. Finally, the report concluded, the decision to transfer patients to Smith-

Mitchell facilities was linked to economic constraints predicated by apartheid structures.

In this regard, reference should be made to the segregation and fragmentation of health services in South Africa. In 1988, the 2.9 billion Rand Public Health Care Budget was split between a bewildering assortment of departments including Own Affairs Ministries, Provincial Administrations, and separate health departments in the self-governing and "independent" homelands (*Financial Mail*, 3 June 1988). According to Freeman from the Community Health Department at the University of the Witwatersrand, mental health facilities were wastefully duplicated under the apartheid system of General and Own Affairs (*The Weekly Mail*, 7–13 June 1991).

The Report of the World Health Organization (1977) found that whereas the majority of White mental patients in South Africa received care in state hospitals and clinics, the vast majority of Black patients received care in inferior private institutions. Moreover, while 17 percent of the White patients were admitted on a voluntary basis, only two percent of Black patients were voluntary patients. The report also found that because privately owned facilities for Black patients operated on a profit-making basis that was dependent on the number of patients detained, and because patients were admitted under involuntary procedures, the system was technically open to abuse. A particular vehicle for abuse lay in the fact that the very same company owning the institutions also owned a drug company, which could lead to a preponderance of use of drugs as opposed to other forms of therapy.

The Society of Psychiatrists of South Africa, in a statement on 8 March 1989, distanced itself from the principle of treating certifiable patients in private institutions (*The Star*, 9 March 1989). It claimed that these institutions could not be classified as hospitals. The head of the Department of Psychiatry at the University of the Witwatersrand, Professor George Hart, said that certifiable patients were "voiceless and unable to stand up for themselves." The Society also noted that although Baragwanath Hospital was one of the southern hemisphere's largest hospitals, it had no inpatient psychiatric ward. Sterkfontein Hospital was the only state-run institution of its type for Black patients on the Witwatersrand.

The South African government spent insufficient funds on those in need of psychiatric care. In 1986, the Department of National Health and Population Development reported a shortage of psychiatric nurses, a lack of funds and personnel, and an increased workload on already overburdened personnel. Because of a lack of adequate facilities, a mentally ill Black child could wait five years before being admitted to an institution, according to Doctor Allwood of Baragwanath Hospital (*The Star*, 25 April 1988). On a research visit made by Vogelman to a Smith-Mitchell institution on the East Rand in the Witwatersrand area in 1986, he found that approximately 500 patients were being tended to by one full-time occupational therapist, one full-time physiotherapist and a few nurses. A medical practitioner and a psychiatrist each consulted at the institution only once a week (Haysom, Strous, & Vogelman, 1990). In the case of the institution mentioned, if the psychiatrist and a psychologist were each to tend to each patient only once a week, this would mean that they would have had to see at least one patient per minute. The Smith-Mitchell institutions' huge standing population of both chronically ill and mentally retarded patients could not derive a reasonable standard of care because of insufficient and overextended staff.

In 1990, the American Association for the Advancement of Science (1990) reported that there were approximately 200 psychiatrists in South Africa to care for a population of approximately 35 million. Of these, only five were Black, Indian, or Colored. A similar disproportionate representation of the race groups could be found in the psychological profession. Most psychiatrists were concentrated in the urban areas and some mental hospitals in the rural areas had no psychiatrists at all.

Allegations of abuse in psychiatric hospitals continued in the early 1990s. In June 1991, the National Medical and Dental Association (NAMDA) called for a Commission of Enquiry into conditions at mental hospitals after allegations were made that Black inmates at the Millsite and Randfontein Sanatoria on the West Rand were malnourished and inadequately clothed, and that there was a high death rate through negligence or winter cold (*The Star*, 7 June 1991). Four years previously, *The Star* newspaper had alleged similar malpractices at the Millsite Sanatorium: an 18-year-old mentally retarded male with epilepsy was found dead by a fellow inmate in a locked garden shed, and one week later a body which had been decomposing for approximately four months had been found under a prefabricated shed. An investigation of the Millsite and Randfontein Sanatoria by *The Weekly Mail* (7–13 June 1991) revealed chronic understaffing, child patients having to share beds, and no crutches or wheelchairs for physically disabled patients. These allegations were denied by both the MEC for Health Services as well as by the Group Managing Director of the Lifecare Group. They stated that the allegations were grossly inaccurate and invited the media to visit facilities. The media perception was of a coverup (*The Weekly Mail*, 14–20 June 1991).

In another incident, after the Transvaal Provincial Administration rejected an application for a visit to Sterkfontein Hospital, a state hospital, staff of *The Weekly Mail* newspaper gained access to the hospital without permission. *The Weekly Mail* (14–20 June 1991) reported that apartheid was rife at the hospital and conditions of treatment depended on one's skin color. The White section near the front of the hospital included a recreation hall, a beauty parlor and clean, well-kept wards. The Black wards, at the back of the premises, had dirty, broken windows and no heating. Patients in Black wards were reported to receive inferior care to patients in the White wards. Health care workers informed journalists of lower patient-staff ratios in White wards and the availability of social workers and psychologists to provide therapy in White wards but not in Black wards. Black patients could apparently be admitted to the White rehabilitation ward on condition that they had a Grade 12 education, spoke English, and could "adapt well to the environment." These requirements did not apply to White patients.

In August 1991, the South African Police were called upon to investigate 18 complaints of assault against a number of nursing personnel at Weskoppies Hospital who allegedly used broomsticks to beat 16 patients. The MEC for Health Services at the Transvaal Provincial Administration stated that staff involved in the incident had been sent on 14 days compulsory leave during the investigations (*The Star*, 6 August 1991). According to figures released in Parliament, at Sterkfontein Hospital alone, 513 patients "escaped, broke out, absconded, or were allowed to go on leave and did not return" between 1986 and 1990 (*The Weekly Mail*, 21–27 June 1991). These incidents and figures highlight the importance of proper management, monitoring, and care of patients, and the range of alleged inadequacies and abuses in the treatment of Black patients.

Administrators have often contested that mistreatment occurs in mental health institutions. However, frequent allegations of human rights violations and allegations of coverups following media exposure need to be understood within the context of racial segregation and inadequate health care for Black patients. Moreover, de facto censoring of information that could be published pertaining to mental institutions raised concerns in the early 1990s as to what was occurring within these institutions.

Mental institutions were treated in the same way as prisons regarding the reporting on their conditions. Section 66A of the Mental Health Act of 1973 cast the onus on any person publishing incorrect information on a mental institution to establish that reasonable steps were taken to verify the truth thereof. An analogous provision in the Prisons Act of 1959 was interpreted in a way that stifled and restricted reporting on prison conditions.

One of the justifications for a provision in the Prisons Act which limited legal supervision of prison conditions was that judges had access to prisons for the purposes of inspecting conditions therein and receiving complaints from prisoners. There was, however, no provision for judges or magistrates to visit mental institutions. Hospital boards were required to visit the institution but it would be doubtful whether a member of a board would have the same authority and stature as a judicial officer (Haysom, Strous & Vogelman, 1990). Haysom et al. contend that the Mental Health Act by medicalizing the committal process undercut the potential for patients to resist confinement and treatment. The monitoring of the treatment of the mentally ill should have been all the more important in that the South African law, unlike that of the United States, did not recognize a clear right of a medical patient to refuse treatment. If, as Ken Owen suggested (*Business Day*, March 1990), patients were "drugged until their condition stabilizes, and then discharged onto the streets" and potential abuses in mental institutions escaped public exposure, those responsible for the decision to commit the mentally ill, notably judges, should at least have been aware of the conditions in mental institutions. Despite a legal veneer, the committal process has been essentially an administrative procedure relying on the diagnosis and opinion of medical practitioners, without adequate safeguards to the human rights of the mentally ill.

SHORTAGES OF MENTAL HEALTH PRACTITIONERS

Services in the public sector, especially for the Black population, have been lamentably inadequate whereas in White, affluent, urban areas, services have been available, accessible and manifestly affordable (Hickson & Kriegler, 1996, p. 153). The state spends little on psychotherapeutic resources in general and the bulk of Black mental patients cannot afford private services (Edelstein, Webber, & Pillay, 1997, p. 135). South Africa's ratio of psychiatrists to seriously incapacitated patients in 1991 was estimated to be 1:1 250, in comparison to 1:190 in Britain and 1:80 in the United States. According to Melvyn Freeman of the Community Health Department at the University of the Witwatersrand, in 1991 only 100 psychologists were state employed, with 20 of them serving a population of about 7 million people in the Black homelands (*The Weekly Mail*, 7–13 June 1991). The ratio of psychiatrists, psychiatric nurses, and social workers to the population has been equally alarming (Freeman, 1992; Freeman & Pillay, 1997).

The bulk of psychiatrists and psychologists are in private practice, estimated to provide care for about 21 percent of the population. This situation has arisen both as a result of there being limited posts in the state and welfare services as well as greater earning potential in the private arena (Edelstein et al., 1997, p. 128). Even when offered a choice, psychologists in the private sector have expressed a preference for private practice (Pillay & Petersen, 1996). In 1996, fewer than 38 percent of psychiatrists registered with the Interim National Medical and Dental Council were employed in the state sector (INMDC, cited by Edelstein et al., 1997). In the same year, fewer than 10 percent of all clinical psychologists in South Africa were public employees.

Private practitioners are usually located in urban areas that are inaccessible to the majority of the population. The majority of professionally trained counselors in South Africa are White, and the services of psychologists and psychiatrists have been primarily situated in the White community (Pillay & Petersen, 1996). In a study conducted by Pillay and Petersen (1996) as to the practice patterns of clinical and counseling psychologists, 92.4 percent of the respondents were White, 2 percent Black, 2.8 percent Indian, and 1 percent Colored. The overwhelming majority of the respondents (91.2 percent) spoke only English or Afrikaans and 80 percent worked exclusively in urban areas. The majority of the respondents (63.3 percent) indicated that over 75 percent of their clients/patients were White, in contrast to only 3.3 percent of respondents who indicated that over 75 percent of their clients/patients were Black. Psychological services in South Africa have been provided mainly by White psychologists and are largely limited to White middle-class patients (Bassa & Schlebusch, 1984; Freeman, 1992; Pillay & Petersen, 1994).

White psychologists are over represented in the profession and the majority of clients/patients with access to clinical and counseling psychologists are drawn from the White minority group. According to Dr Saths Cooper, a past president of the Psychological Society of South Africa, 85 percent of South African psychologists are White (Cavill, 2000).

Private practitioners have limited training and experience in dealing with cultural, social, and language contexts of disadvantaged communities. Moreover, therapy processes may be substantially compromised by therapist ignorance of Black languages or the need for an interpreter (L. Swartz, 1998).

Advantages offered by the private sector are its flexibility as well as the accountability of each practitioner (Edelstein et al., 1997). However, private practitioners may be motivated by profit motifs and may neglect costly prevention programs. While the private sector offers a broad range of psychotherapeutic services, the ceiling placed on annual benefits payable by medical aid schemes means that for many South Africans only a limited number of sessions are affordable. Individual therapy is unable to meet the needs of the mass of the population (Psychological Association of South Africa, 1989). Richter et al. (1998) have advocated for the establishment of psychology within all sectors of the civil service as the only way to ensure access for all South Africans to a broad range of social and psychological services available in the profession. That psychology in South Africa is a predominantly private practice profession is contrary to the rights and redress agendas currently guiding service development in the country (Richter et al., 1998, p. 6).

RACISM IN SOUTH AFRICAN PSYCHOLOGY

Although psychology is frequently considered a liberal humanity, the psychological terrain in South Africa has a long racist past (Foster, 1991, p. 206). South

African psychology has viewed its society through the distorted lens of racial pathology and has often lent its skills and talents in the actualization of racist visions (Cooper et al., 1990). The term "servants of apartheid" (Webster, 1981) has at times been aptly fitting for some psychological activities in South Africa (Foster, Nicholas, & Dawes, 1993).

The Truth and Reconciliation Commission (TRC) found that in South Africa the area of mental health has been historically neglected. It noted that care has been predominantly institutional, there are few trained psychologists and social workers, and few attempts have been made to provide culturally appropriate mental health care to all South Africans. In a consideration of the consequences of gross violations of human rights during the apartheid years, the Commission noted suspicions that diagnoses of mental illness were used to silence activists or opponents by condemning them to institutions where they were under state control. Mental health professionals are alleged to have advised torturers on how to identify potential victims, break down their resistance and exploit their vulnerabilities. This contributed to resistance to seeking formal psychological treatment. The TRC Report also cited difficulty in obtaining appropriate services where these were sought.

Psychology as a separate discipline was established in South Africa in the 1920s, a time when the imagery of Social Darwinism was discernible in three areas of political debate: racial differences in intelligence, the widespread "horror" of miscegenation, and fears of racial and moral degeneration (Dubow, 1987; Foster, 1993). Foster (1991a, 1991b, 1993) has linked the promotion of racism in South Africa to two eminent psychologists: H.F. Verwoerd and W.A. Willemse. Verwoerd completed Masters and Doctoral degrees at the University of Stellenbosch and in 1927 was appointed the first Professor of Applied Psychology at the university. He took up Afrikaner sectionalist interests, became involved in the poor White problem, opposed immigration by Jewish refugees from Nazi Germany, and became a chief architect of apartheid and Prime Minister of South Africa. Willemse, who obtained a Psychology Doctorate from Pretoria in 1929, also became a leading figure in the development of Afrikaner nationalism and racist thinking. He was a close colleague of Geoff Cronje, a key ideologue of 1940s race thinking. In 1942, Willemse proposed a system of racial classification for the population as a whole. He contended that Blacks were both culturally and intellectually inferior and he opposed "race-mixing."

Other psychologists whose work contributed to racist views were Malherbe, Wilcocks, and Van Schalkwyk. They promoted upliftment of the poor White population, effectively neglecting the question of Black poverty. Wilcocks advocated for the revision and extension of legislation aimed at keeping racial groups apart and at ensuring the perpetual domination of Whites. He canvassed for the deprivation of work opportunities for Blacks. He also called for legislation to inflict severe penalties on interracial sexual intercourse (Cooper et al., 1990; Wilcocks, 1932). Psychiatrists such as Dunstan and Laubscher also advocated racist views (Foster, 1993).

In accordance with Verwoerd's insistence as Prime Minister on racial segregation in South African society, the Psychological Institute of the Republic of South Africa (PIRSA), a group that had broken away from the South African Psychological Association, excluded Blacks from membership of the society (Wortley, 2000). Leading members of PIRSA were members of the secret Afrikaner Broederbond. Some PIRSA members attempted to develop psychological theory compatible with the apartheid regime's prevailing Christian Nationalist perspective. PIRSA President,

A.J. la Grange referred to "a natural need for self protection against a world wide hysterical mass movement of equalization" (cited by Foster, 1991). In 1967, PIRSA President-elect, P.M. Robbertse, commented favorably on research into race differences in intelligence, called for further such work, cited evidence of Blacks' inferior brain size, and referred to fascist journals and sympathizers in a display of blatant and crude racism (Foster, 1993).

In 1982, the Psychological Association of South Africa (PASA) was formed. This organization generally sided with the status quo. It failed to provide unequivocal condemnation of political detention and mental health abuses of the apartheid system, used apartheid-oriented language, and attempted to break the antiapartheid academic boycott (Foster et al., 1993).

POSITIVIST AND ACONTEXTUAL RESEARCH

South African psychology's collusion, both active and tacit, with apartheid systems and human rights violations did not greatly compromise its local or international scientific standing. Raubenheimer (1993) felt comfortable suggesting in *The Psychologist*, the official bulletin of the British Psychological Society, that criticisms of psychology's role in Africa (Akin-Ogundeji, 1991) were not pertinent to South African psychology, which was flourishing both academically professionally.

If psychology is never separate from its host culture (Richards, 1997, p. 153), how was it possible for South African psychology to uphold its credibility internationally and locally when apartheid was being defined as an international crime against humanity? A large part of the answer resides in psychology's adherence to the rigors of supposedly value-free empirical research (Biesheuwel, 1987). Many South African psychologists adopted a "scientific" and medical view of psychology, rejecting accusations of racism by insisting on their even-handed proficiency at scientific and medical practice (Durrheim & Mokeki, 1997).

The lack of a critical social focus in South African psychology was exonerated by the discipline's supposed status as a value-free science. Positivist methodology, which has predominated in South African psychological research (Durrheim & Mokeki, 1997; Seedat, 1997; Whittle, 1985), has as its main concern the importation of the methodology of the natural sciences into social studies in order to avoid the contaminating effects of research bias. This approach insists that science must be logical, objective, value-free and empirical, distinguishing between facts of what "is" and normative statements of what "ought" to be.

The value-free science model of psychology underlies an overwhelming concern with developing knowledge and technology without regarding their functions in society (Durrheim & Mokeki, 1997). This uncritical stance has unwittingly served political interests. By intentionally ignoring value judgments, mainstream positivist approaches fail to challenge the status quo and may tacitly incorporate its values. Strauss (1975) puts it that positivists fiddle while Rome burns; which is excused by two facts—they neither know that they fiddle nor that Rome burns (p. 344).

Positivists generally have a consensual understanding of society in which behavioral norms are taken as being agreed upon by the majority of the population. An act that "could possibly be justified from the standpoint of an alternative view of social morality" (Heather, 1976, p. 104) may be dismissed as evidence of individual maladjustment. The implications of positivist assumptions are, according to Young (1981), that a deviant "would be a rule breaker in any culture—a pacifist during wartime, and an aggressor during peace." There is no attempt to explain the content of norms that are violated, but merely the propensity of the individual to violate them.

In some instances, positivist methodology has led to tacit support for iniquitous regimes. It has appealed also to those actively supportive of the status quo. Under the ambit of "value-free science," South African psychology has done much to actively support apartheid and racism, propagating racist stereotypes and conducting pro-apartheid research (Durrheim & Mokeki, 1997; Cooper & Nicholas, 1990).

The major racist implications of the positivist tradition is the imposition of dominant values on members of disempowered groups. Crude positivism follows an etic trend; assuming a culturally universal or generalized model of mental health. Behavior is interpreted regardless of social context. This is in opposition to an emic approach, which regards behavioral interpretations as valid only when referred to a person's indigenous cultural norms.

Adherence to a noncritical, conservative ideology at a time when apartheid adversely affected the mental well being of most South Africans through its generation of stress situations brings into question psychology's scientific or moral respectability (Dawes, 1985). The call for psychology to remain professionally neutral so as to not compromise itself as a profession (Biesheuvel, 1987; Van Aarde, 1987) was curious given its accompaniment by direct political announcements and advocacy of social engineering in the service of apartheid (Nicholas, 1990, 1993).

African psychological research by Euro-American psychologists has largely echoed the racist, ethnocentric, and class biases of colonial and imperialistic interests (Bulhan, 1993). There is a paucity of research systematically examining:

1. the historical development of psychology within an apartheid framework;
2. programs, trends, and silences within the field; and nuances around the exclusion and marginalization of Blacks and women from the process and generation of knowledge,
3. production and accreditation in the field itself (Seedat, 1997).

Editorial policies in South African psychology journals have tended to render Black scholars voiceless and powerless in the domain of knowledge production by failing to speak out and deal with racialized patterns of research and authorship reflected in their journals (Duncan, 1998). According to Duncan, disparities between Black and White authorship illustrate psychology's complicity in academic racism.

Academics who "publish or perish" have had to submit to constraining publication criteria of objectivity and neutrality within a decontextualized, positivist framework (Seedat, 1997). Articles published in the *South African Journal of Psychology*, the official journal of the Psychological Association of South Africa (subsequently reconstituted as PsySSA), between 1983 and 1988, were predominantly "empirical in nature, devoid of any social and theoretical relevance to the oppressed majority in South Africa" (Seedat, 1997, p. 29). South African psychologists seldom undertook to research significant national problems during the years 1981 to 1984 (Whittle, 1985). In fact, an analysis by Durrheim and Mokeki of all papers published in the *South African Journal of Psychology* between 1970 and 1995 shows a pronounced dip in papers that critically considered racial issues during the early 1980s. This was a time of intense political struggle and violent repression in South Africa, yet psychologists could "legitimately" ignore issues of race by cleaving to medical and "value-free" models of psychology (Durrheim & Mokeki, 1997). Cooper and Nicholas (1990) state that more foreign than South African psychologists articulated the psychological consequences of apartheid.

The quest for a liberatory psychology, transformation, and emancipation, may be stifled in the names of scientific neutrality and objectivity (Seedat, 1997). The implication of positions antagonistic to positivism is that real needs in times of stress must take preference over the pursuance of scientific purity, and social scientists must put their knowledge to the service of social and political change (Easton, 1971). To be relevant, South African psychologists need to venture out of ivory towers of "neutral" research and commit themselves to meaningful social change.

Cloete and Pillay (1988) contend that intellectuals serve their own interests and those of the order to which they are aligned through silence, as a "containment of critical energy" (Disco, 1979, p. 168). White elites are implicated in everyday racism through passivity, acquiescence, ignorance, and indifference regarding ethnic or racial inequality and through condoning or refraining from action against the discursive reproduction of racism (Van Dijk, 1993).

Many psychologists, already socialized within the cultural milieu of a White-centered, racist society, would have been inducted in South Africa into a profession which largely neglected to research contextual injustices, was over reliant on positivist assumptions and methodology, and excluding of Black opinions. Psychologists who romanticize the virtues of their discipline as a science are, as stated by Manganyi (1991), in need of a good dose of "historical realism." South African psychology has certainly been largely "ensconced within the legacy of colonialism, apartheid and patriarchy" (Seedat, 1998, p. 83).

SITES OF RESISTANCE

A focus on psychology's collusion in acontextualized conservatism and racial discrimination would be too monolithic an approach without reference to sites of resistance and efforts to ensure an alternative, racism-free society. It is possible to find a lever for change only through attention to contradiction and working through spaces of resistance opened up by competing accounts and alternative practices (Parker, 1999, p. 4). South African and international history is replete with evidence of struggles of resistance against racism and apartheid (Nkomo et al., 1995). In the field of psychology, progressively minded psychologists to the left of the political mainstream, who identified with the struggle for a nonracial democracy in South Africa, tried to address themselves to the structural determinants of problems experienced in the South African apartheid system and its aftermath, and articulated the need to place psychology in its wider socio-economic, political, racial, and cultural context (e.g., Cloete, Pillay & Swartz, 1986; Dawes, 1985; Hayes, 1986; Ivey, 1986; Lambley, 1980; Swartz & Foster, 1984; Swartz, Dowdall, & Swartz, 1986; Turton, 1986).

The establishment of the Organization for Appropriate Social Services in South Africa (OASSSA) is illustrative of attempts made to provide appropriate mental health and social services in a manner consistent with the political goals of the progressive movement. Two fundamental principles of OASSSA were:

1. A focus on the provision of services for those suffering under the yoke of apartheid, be it from detention, economic exploitation, political oppression or any other such process; and

2. An alignment in a nonsectarian manner with the progressive movement (Flisher, Skinner, Lazarus, & Louw, 1993).

In terms of research, *Psychology in South Africa (PINS)* established itself as a journal concerned about "the uses and abuses to which 'psychology' is put in the maintenance of apartheid and other forms of social oppression" (Editorial, August 1984). The journal attracted many papers criticizing the decontextualised and desocialised notions of psychological theory and practice, and dealing with pertinent social topics (Seedat, 1990).

OASSSA and *PINS* represent two well-recognized attempts to challenge the role of psychology in the apartheid system, and there were others. Nevertheless, these attempts were not part of the prevailing mainstream. Mainstream psychology focused on positivist premises of neutrality and political noninvolvement. The progressive movement provided an intellectual and professional space for South African counselors and therapists to question the ruling hegemony, but the real impetus for counselor sensitivity to the needs of disempowered individuals and groups probably derives as much from multicultural counseling theory as it does from the political left.

SUMMARY

In the area of mental health, racial discrimination resulted in facilities for Blacks that were inadequate compared to those for Whites. Mental asylums in South Africa were racially segregated and have been criticized as providing inferior standards of care for Black patients. In addition, there have been insufficient safeguards against human rights violations in such institutions. Moreover, while counseling services in the public sector are inadequate for the majority Black population, private services are largely available, accessible, and affordable in traditionally White urban areas.

In the main, the practice and study of psychology flourished within the institutions and ideology of apartheid. The involvement of psychologists in segregated school services, which upheld apartheid teachings, in industry to entrench unequal power relations, and in professional organizations that excluded Blacks, brings into question psychology's stance on racial exploitation and the struggle for change (Cooper et al., 1990). Although psychology is frequently considered a liberal humanity, it has a long racist past in South Africa. Racist psychologists supported and propagated the apartheid vision, and some are alleged to have even engaged actively in supporting human rights abuses. These activities and the lack of a critical social focus in South African psychology were exonerated by the discipline's status as a self-portrayed value-free science. Today, psychology's scientific and moral respectability are at stake because of its collusion, be it active or tacit, in oppression.

3

Counselor Encapsulation

ENCAPSULATION

Counselors who are encapsulated may be considered to be protected in their own environments, removed largely from the psychosocial experiences that affect many of their potential clients, and with a truncated appreciation of factors informing client worldviews. Therapists are often not prepared to deal with clients from racial, ethnic, or socio-economic groups whose values, attitudes, and general lifestyle differ from White middle-class norms (Gordon, 1965; Locke & Lewis, 1969; Padilla, Boxley & Wagner, 1972). Cultural, class, race, and language differences may hinder therapy; and counselors intent on establishing therapeutic rapport and effectively handling client-therapist alliances and transference-countertransference phenomena face extra challenges in interracial and multicultural contexts.

Wrenn (1962) wrote of the potential for counselors in a rapidly changing world to become encapsulated in their own worlds, culture, and worldview, a danger he referred to as "cultural encapsulation." Cultural encapsulation refers to the protective capsule or cocoon that some counselors construct to protect themselves from meaningful engagement with persons from other cultures. Counselors who disregard cultural variations among clients and dogmatically adhere to technique-oriented notions of universal truth may be said to be "culturally encapsulated" (Wrenn, 1962; Pedersen, 1976).

The following features of cultural encapsulation have been identified by Wrenn (1985, cited by Pedersen, 1997):

1. A definition of reality according to one's own set of cultural assumptions.
2. Insensitivity to the cultural variations of others and the assumption that one's own view is right.
3. The truth of cultural assumptions is accepted without scrutiny, even despite contrary evidence.
4. Solutions are sought through technique-oriented job definitions and quick or simple remedies.
5. A self-reference criterion is used to evaluate others' viewpoints regardless of their cultural context (p. 32).

The notion of cultural encapsulation is somewhat controversial, especially in the South African context, because of a tendency to conflate culture and "race." Arguments of cultural deficiency may mask real racism. Recent descriptions of multiculturalism and counselor sensitivity (e.g., 1991, 1997) emphasize the importance of nondomination and respect of differences. However, calls from within the multicultural movement for the amelioration of cultural encapsulation could inadvertently contribute to the conflation of "race" and culture and cultural racism by unaware counselors.

As Ponterotto and Pedersen (1993, p. 7) point out, the term "culture" has often been used synonymously with "race" in the counseling literature. This has also happened in political talk. In South Africa, "cultural difference" was used as a discursive construct to advocate separation of the races and White privilege. In reality, not all Black people are part of one culture and not all White people are part of one culture. However, as stated by Wetherell and Potter (1992):

Culture has this aura of niceness, of progressiveness and humanitarianism. It covers over the messy business of domination and uneven development through advocacy of respect and tolerance for differences. Colonial history can be reconstructed as a story of clashing values, the modern against the traditional, as opposed to a story of conflicting interests, power relations and exploitation. There is an inevitability and acceptability in the notion of "culture contact" not found in the rhetoric of annexation, conquest and oppression. (p. 137)

The culturalization of racism emerged through the justification of racial inequality as a function of cultural difference and the need to preserve the *Other's* culture (Essed, 1987). Essed (1991) contends that: "The norm of cultural tolerance legitimizes objectification of Blacks for Whites to control the nature and extent of cultural differences. The language of tolerance expresses goodwill, while the practice of tolerance means that other cultures are scrutinized, categorized, labeled, and assessed by dominant norms and values" (p. 211).

The term "counselor encapsulation," which is frequently used interchangeably with the term "cultural encapsulation," may better serve to describe the conceptual separation of culture and "race," without losing the connotation of a limitation of perspective. Counselor encapsulation involves substituting stereotypes for the real world in a way that allows counselors to evade reality, and which brings into question the effectiveness and credibility of counseling services. Traditionally trained counselors frequently assume that existing counseling theories and techniques are appropriate for all people, regardless of their race, ethnicity, or culture. Their assumption that they are equipped with skills equally applicable for all populations, no matter how diverse, means that in some respects their training is a liability (Ridley, 1995).

There have been calls for psychologists to be: "constantly mindful not only of the subtle ways in which they may perpetuate racism in their work—theorizing, research, writings and practice—but also the ways in which they are recruited and trained to do the dirty work, as it were, of those with a vested interest in the status quo" (Owusu & Bempah-Howitt, 1999, p. 139).

Well-intentioned therapists may be unaware that they are behaving in racist ways because they have been socialized in racist societies in which the ideology of racism is largely unquestioned. Unintentional or covert racism is unlikely to be challenged because of a lack of awareness on the part of the actor of wrong-doing (Pedersen, 1977, p. 31).

WORLDVIEW

In addition to counselor encapsulation, another useful term that relates to the need to broaden personal perspectives in order to understand others is that of "worldview." Worldview refers to the manner in which people perceive their relationships to nature, institutions, other people, and things (D.W. Sue, 1979,1979b). Sluzki (1983) recognizes that we all carry within ourselves "Weltanschauungen," belief structures that are based on assumptions, some of which are clearly crystallized into ideologies, some into convictions, and many more that fuse conceptions and preconceptions into "that is the way things are."

"One cannot not have a world view (which is, of course, a world view)" (Sluzki, 1983, p. 472). Worldview is correlated with cultural background, socio-political history, and life experiences. It constitutes psychological orientation in life and can determine cognitive and behavioral patterns, decision making, and how events are defined (Hickson & Kriegler, 1996). Interacting components influencing a person's worldview may include race, ethnicity, age, life stage, lifestyle, gender, social class, degree of acculturation, education, ordinal position in family, marital status, and geographical locale (Hickson & Kriegler, 1996).

An understanding and respect of worldview in counseling clients of different backgrounds has a number of advantages:

1. It assists counselors in understanding both their clients and themselves.
2. It makes explicit both the counselor's and client's values, beliefs, suppositions and attributions.
3. It facilitates the choice of mutually agreed-upon goals and processes appropriate to the client.
4. It provides the subjective reality that is important in gaining knowledge and developing meaningful skills.
5. It enhances ethical counseling by making counselors aware of imposing culturally dominant beliefs, paternalism, condescension, and mislabeling clients as "sick" (Caylef, 1986; Hickson, Christie & Shmukler, 1990; Ibrahim & Arrendondo, 1986).

Ethnocentric strategies, which ignore worldview, may produce conflict and militate against trust and an effective therapeutic alliance. Therapy training frequently presents White middle-class, urban, English-speaking, traditionally structured values as a normative measure. Given the massive power difference between therapists and clients of different backgrounds, the potential for ineffectual interaction is great. Most of the therapeutic goals in therapy have been toward establishing normative behaviors in a middle-class dominant society. A therapeutic awareness that includes an understanding of social stratification, cultural expectations and value systems, rather than only family or personal pathology, is required (Axelson, 1985; Boynton, 1987; Day, 1983; Ho, 1987; Kaplan, 1971; Lau, 1984; Maranhão, 1984; McGoldrick, 1982). An understanding of clients' worldviews in relation to the therapist's is probably a vital ingredient for therapeutic success.

Both clients and counselors may feel disturbed due to variations between their own perspectives and the values and perspectives of the other party in a therapy dyad. While Raubenheimer (1993) suggested that many Blacks might struggle to adapt to and keep abreast of ever-changing demands in the workplace, Foster et al. (1993) predicted that more Whites than Blacks might find it bewildering to adapt to changes in South Africa. White clinicians, schooled, socialized, and trained in ways that cocooned them from the multicultural, socioeconomic, and racial realities of South Africa, have held and are still likely to hold distorted or inadequate knowledge of diverse client worldviews and therapy preferences.

EUROCENTRIC ASSUMPTIONS

A common feature of psychoanalysis and client-centered counseling is that they proffer Northern Hemisphere, Western technocentric rationales as universally and transhistorically applicable techniques (Pilgrim, 1997). The innovators of these techniques have been disparagingly dubbed "DWEMs" (Dead, White, European Males) by feminists; and the term "DWAMs" (Dead, White, American, Males) could be added, comments Pilgrim in an equivalently disparaging tone (p. 80).

Hussein Bulhan (1985, 1990) has criticized Eurocentric psychology as solipsistic; that is, as having a perspective that only the "self" exists or continues to exist. According to Bulhan, the majority of Africans explain health or illness, diagnosis or treatment in relational rather than intrapsychic terms. Afrocentric psychology is systemic and relational rather than individualistic, states Bulhan. He has called upon South African psychologists to liberate themselves from the framework of solipsism, which, he charges, permeates Eurocentric psychology.

In the United States, Vickie Mays (1985, p. 380) contends that White psychology ignores the fact that although slavery and institutional racism attempted to strip Black Americans of their culture and identity, the remnants of African philosophy help Black Americans to survive and define what mental health is. The promulgation of a White model of mental health is a form of intolerance, which effectively denies Black Americans' ethnic identity.

American and European counseling have frequently presumed "an individualistic perspective in which dependency is always bad, privacy is universally valued, and the welfare of each individual is always more important than the value of the group to which the individual belongs. In the global, more typically collective context this perspective is exotic and extraordinary" (Pedersen & Leong, 1997, p. 119).

According to Hickson and Kriegler (1996), the White minority in South Africa has stressed Eurocentric values of the primacy of the individual over the group, materialism, competition, self-interest, independence, privacy, and assertiveness. An Afrocentric worldview, in contrast, stresses a group ethic, collective good, unity of the universe, and the notion that spirit and matter are one.

Eurocentric Assumptions and Diagnosis

The detrimental effects of counselor encapsulation apply not only to the counseling process but also to diagnostic and prognostic formulations, which in Western practice frequently precede and influence counseling. A number of studies suggest that therapeutic effectiveness depends on formulative predictions as to the cause of illness, obstacles to therapy, motivation, and patient resources and defenses (Swartz, 1999, p. 45).

In the field of psychodynamic theory and practice, for instance, issues as basic as definitions of selfhood, experience of self in time, and values around separation-individuation may be specific to Western middle-class society (Bracero, 1994). When it was originally formulated, psychoanalysis, which has had a profound impact on how Westerners think about emotional dysfunction, was based on a patient-physician bond which did not take into account cultural or social differences between patients and doctors, such as different diagnostic explanations and procedures, because doctors and patients came from essentially the same social milieu (Littlewood & Lipsedge, 1997, p. 56). The raising of questions of cultural difference by the patient was interpreted as a form of therapy resistance. Given this disregard of social context, ethnic minorities and colonized societies were able to be perceived as child-like in therapeutic contexts, and the relations of colonial psychiatrist and colonized individual were perceived in parent-child terms. Thus, Jung could postulate Negroes to have "a whole layer less" of cultural strata and warned that "living with barbaric races exerts a suggestive effect on the laboriously tamed instinct of the white race and tends to pull it down" (Thomas & Sillen, cited by Littlewood & Lipsedge, p. 56).

A consistent theme in clinical literature is that Blacks or ethnic minorities are more likely to receive a diagnosis of serious and longstanding mental disorder or psychosis than are Whites (Strebel, Msomi & Stacey, 1999, p. 54). Blacks are less likely to be diagnosed as suffering from mood disorders and are more likely to be diagnosed as schizophrenic, especially paranoid schizophrenic, or as suffering from an organic disorder, than are Whites. Many writers argue that Blacks are over-pathologized when it comes to clinical diagnosis, and that they receive harsher psychiatric forms of treatment than do Whites (Littlewood & Lipsedge, 1997).

Swartz (1998) draws attention to the Diagnostic and Statistical Manual of Mental Disorders (Fourth Edition) (DSM-IV) of the American Psychiatric Association, which states that when it comes to classifying symptoms, in addition to other diagnostic criteria, reference should be made to the following cultural factors:

1. The cultural identity of the individual.
2. Cultural explanations of the individual's illness.
3. Cultural factors related to psychosocial environment and level of functioning.
4. Cultural elements of the relationship between the individual and the clinician.
5. Overall cultural assessment for diagnosis and care (The Diagnostic and Statistical Manual of Mental Disorders Fourth Edition [DSM-IV], 1994, pp. 843–844).

A clinician who is unfamiliar with the nuances of an individual's frame of reference may incorrectly judge as psychopathology those normal variations in behavior, belief, or experience that are particular to the individual's culture. For example, certain religious practices or beliefs (for example, hearing or seeing a deceased relative during bereavement) may be misdiagnosed as manifestations of a Psychotic Disorder. Applying Personality Disorder criteria across cultural settings may be especially difficult because of the wide cultural variation in concepts of self, styles of communication, and coping mechanisms (DSM-IV, 1994).

According to Leslie Swartz (1998), African indigenous healing differs from Western taxonomies not only in terms of actual labels and diagnoses given, but also in terms of how diagnostic systems are constructed. Diagnosis in African indigenous healing may be better understood as related to theories of causation or illness rather than simply to authoritative taxonomies such as the Manual of the American Psychiatric Association, DSM-IV, or ICD-10, its World Health Organization equivalent. African ideas about causation of illness relate to a range of issues in the natural, social, personal, spiritual, and political realms, states Swartz (1998). *Amafufunyana*, for example, a form of spirit possession or hysteria occurring amongst Zulu and Xhosa-speakers, may have different diagnostic features in different contexts. Divisions between mind and body and between assessment and treatment tend to be less rigid in African indigenous healing than in DSM-IV. In African indigenous healing, the process of healing itself—which may involve drumming and dancing—can provide more information about the problem as treatment proceeds. (There is some similarity here to client-centered approaches, which value the healing relationship above diagnostic acumen (Holdstock, 1981a; Swartz, 1998). A heavy reliance on contextual hermeneutics in African indigenous healing distinguishes it from DSM-IV, which tries to be context-free (Swartz, 1998).

Diagnostic activity based on DSM-IV criteria tends to look for pathology in order to name it (Combrink-Graham, 1987). This often tends to result in evaluative descriptions of malfunction (Dell, 1985). Ecosystemically oriented thinking, in contrast, focuses on a nonpejorative explanation of how a system works. As already noted with reference to Eurocentric psychology, and of particular relevance to diagnosis, Afrocentric psychology may follow a more relational and systemic as opposed to a solipsistic appreciation (Bulhan, 1990). Traditional African approaches are less exclusively self-referenced and tend to encompass a more interactive system than Western psychodynamic formulations (Gumede, 1990; Hammond-Tooke, 1989; Straker, 1994).

According to Leslie Swartz (1998), the major focus of African healing is on *ukufu Kwabantu* ("diseases of the African people"). In African indigenous healing, illness may be attributed to a range of contextual issues such as ecological imbalance, pollution, impaired social relationships, bewitchment, or sorcery (because of jealousy or for other reasons), or through disturbed relationships with the spiritual world—such as not complying with the wishes of ancestors. In contrast, emphasis on the cultural is to be found only at the peripheries of Western diagnostic systems (Swartz, 1998).

Leslie Swartz (1998) cites a study by Rumble and her colleagues as an example of a Western classification system leading to misdiagnosis in South Africa. Rumble et al. (1996) found exceptionally high rates of psychosis in a South African community. On re-examining their data, they factored in that blaming others for misfortune, including believing that one is bewitched, is a culturally appropriate explanation for misfortune in that community. The rate of diagnosis of psychosis dropped and that of depression increased.

In historical Western psychiatric literature, depression has typically been viewed as rare among "nonEuropeans" (Littlewood & Lipsedge, 1997). Nowadays, there is a changing perception that depression in Africa may be more prevalent (Swartz, 1998). In fact, depression may be even more prevalent in Africa than in Western countries (Dhadphale, M., Ellison, R., & Griffin, L; Odejide et al., 1989; Orley & Wing, 1979; Rwegellera & Mambwe, 1977). Littlewood and Lipsedge (1997, p. 68), and Swartz (1998, p. 111) argue that in the context of few psychiatric facilities, only people with socially disruptive behavior are likely to receive attention. Depressed people whose problems do not seem extreme may be reluctant to seek help when clinical facilities are inadequate. Nondetection of depression may thus reflect the biases and political agenda of Western medicine.

In addition to the under diagnosis of depression in Africa, there has been a common worldwide perception that Blacks somatize more than Whites (Littlewood & Lipsedge, 1997). It is commonly accepted in the West that somatic presentation of distress is an "unsophisticated" phenomenon associated with "less developed" societies. However, throughout the world, including the Western World, there is evidence that using the body to speak of and experience distress is more common than experiencing distress and anxiety in purely psychological terms (Abas et al., 1995; Kleinman, 1986; L. Swartz, 1998). The emergence of chronic fatigue syndrome which affects many successful, middle-class Westerners and which has attracted considerable debate as to its causes and nature, is a case in point. Its appearance in DSM-IV as "undifferentiated somatoform disorder" has helped raise questions about an evolutionist view of somatization (Swartz, 1998).

Western professionals' own ideas about somatization interact with, and are influenced by, more general beliefs about race, culture, and sophistication (L. Swartz, 1991, 1998). Clients from disempowered groups who present with somatic complaints may be negatively stereotyped by Western medicine, which emphasizes a mind-body dichotomy. From a less disparaging perspective, rather than being regarded as a medical syndrome, somatization may be considered a language, a way of seeing the world and engaging with it, so that meanings and social problems are translated into individual processes of communication and attention (Lewis-Fernandez & Kleinman, 1995). The expression of emotional distress in bodily terms has, however, provided a rationale for nonservice delivery by ethnocentric mental health professionals. Jenkins and Valiente (1994) argue that there is a traditional dualist idea that the closer we come to the body the further away we must be from culture: "Long-standing dualisms of the mind as cultural and the body as biological have often served to render the physical, sensational world of pangs, vapours and twinges theoretically insignificant and largely absent from cultural-symbolic analysis" (p 164, cited in Swartz, 1998, p. 143).

An understanding of complaints as neither exclusively physical nor exclusively emotional would permit investigation of how an experiential embodiment of contextual distress interacts with healing systems (Swartz, 1998). Ideologically encapsulated counselors may ignore this process and impose a mind-body dualism on clients who perceive their complaints differently.

Swartz (1998) has provided a comprehensive review of South African cultural factors pertaining to depression, somatization, transient psychosis, schizophrenia, posttraumatic stress disorder, alcohol and drug use, and "culture bound syndromes" such as *amafufunyana* and *ukuthwasa* (emotional turmoil experienced on the path to becoming an indigenous healer, but with additional connotations as well). Swartz concludes, *inter alia*, that we ought "to think about some of the lessons that a cultural understanding can give us towards reaching the ambitious goal of better mental health for all" (1998, p. 244).

In a study of hospital records of patients admitted to three public psychiatric hospitals in the Western Cape for a calendar year (Strebel, Msomi, & Stacey, 1999), consistently significant differences in psychiatric diagnosis and management across race and gender were found, reflecting past inequalities of South African society. Based on their findings, the researchers recommended that:

1. Further epidemiological research is required to investigate issues of reliability and validity in psychiatric diagnosis and practice in South Africa, particularly with regard to sexist and racist bias.
2. Such research also needs to consider the mechanisms whereby social factors interact with other etiological processes to impact on mental health.
3. Psychiatric practice based almost exclusively on dominant Western conceptualizations needs to be challenged.
4. Existing and new mental health workers need to be trained to respond appropriately to language and cultural diversity. (Strebel, Msomi, & Stacey, 1999).

In summary, there is much to suggest that differences between Western and African diagnostic practices may lead to misunderstanding. If psychology is to be accessible and usable by all South Africans, diagnostic procedures and assumptions will need to be revisited. Practitioners are going to have to review their diagnostic assumptions and procedures for reliability, validity and fairness. As Pedersen and Leong (1997) state: "The most dangerous assumption of all is to assume that we already know all our assumptions" (p. 119).

AFROCENTRIC HEALING AS A RESOURCE

According to the National Department of Health estimates in 1997, at least 80 percent of Black South Africans consult traditional healers (Bodibe & Sodi, 1997). Sangomas, sorcerers, herbalists, diviners and faith healers are amongst traditional healers who form a full part of the socio-cultural life of many communities (Buhrmann, 1977). Hickson and Kriegler (1996) have pointed to a perfect match between indigenous healers and Africa's communal system, which occurs through the healer's participation in communal life and the community's participation in the healing process.

Up until the recent past, traditional healing was officially frowned upon and marginalized because it was perceived to be based on mystical and magical religious beliefs (Hopa, Simbaya & du Toit, 1998). Despite official positions taken by the new African National Congress government, calls for an integration of indigenous African and Western health systems (e.g., Buhrmann, 1983; Thabede, 1991) have not yet been realized. Bodibe and Sodi (1997) outline the following requirements for psychologists to meaningfully explore indigenous healing:

1. Extricating ourselves from conceptual complacency and being prepared to commute mentally between dominant Western paradigms and neglected indigenous models.
2. Acknowledging that cultural and personal similarity between healers and clients leads to more effective counseling and psychotherapy.
3. Not treating traditional healers as obstacles to good mental health care.
4. Recognizing that accepted Western methods of psychology and psychiatry, when transported holus bolus to Africa, can have serious limitations (p. 184).

ACCULTURATION

The discussion of counselor encapsulation has thus far focused on the limitation of perspective that may make it difficult for White counselors to appreciate the worldviews of their Black patients. The content of Eurocentric and of Afrocentric diagnostic systems and practices have been discussed and compared. However, it is important to note that not all White counselors necessarily adhere to discretely defined notions of mental health and not all Black clients adhere rigidly to strictly Afrocentric systems. The availability of resources, levels of cultural identity, class issues, and racial identity levels are some factors that may influence choices.

Swartz (1998) cautions against an oversimplified expectation that users of health services choose only those services that seem to share their worldview. Frequently, people have to use what is available rather than their first choice. Moreover, there are many and contradictory worldviews in South Africa, not just one or two. It is not possible to provide a Western service for Western people and a nonWestern service for nonWestern people. The categories "Western" and "non-Western," points out Swartz (p. 92), "are our own creations, and reflect neither the diversity of beliefs (often mutually contradictory) that people hold, nor the commonalities that exist across apparently very different groups of people" (Boonzaaier & Sharp, 1988; Swartz, 1998).

Clients who are living in more than one culture often experience a sense of allegiance to their culture of origin while being attracted to aspects of a new or alternative culture. Cultural change in any form is often a difficult process (Brislin, 1981) and may lead to inner and social conflict. Africans adapting to Western systems may experience a disturbing psycho-existential crisis (Bulhan, 1980).

Clients' difficulties in integrating different cultural influences need to be acknowledged (Pedersen, 1988). Clients may experience acculturative stress in their everyday lives as well as within the therapy milieu, resulting in identity confusion, psychopathology, lowered mental health status, confusion, anxiety, depression, feelings of alienation, and heightened psychosomatic symptoms. South African psychologists need to be especially sensitive to processes of acculturation for their clients who stand central within the country's transitional process (Nortier & Theron, 1998). Counselor sensitivity to acculturative processes requires counselors to arrive at an appreciation and acceptance of how they themselves have been socialized into different cultural norms and practices, and how these norms and practices may interact with those of their clients.

THE IMPACT OF CLASS

Social class is an important variable increasingly foregrounded in counseling literature. A criticism of cross-cultural psychology is that it has neglected important issues of race as well as of class and power imbalances (Vogelman, 1986). A tendency to perceive culture as a pure essence may obscure the impact of political processes, social class, communities' self-definitions, and dynamics of cultural transformation (Seedat, 1990). An historical and materialist analysis of existing services has been called for to facilitate the development of appropriate training, practice, and research which reflect the interests of the broader society and not just a middle-class bourgeois elite (Dawes, 1986).

Attitudes about social class may function to exaggerate stereotypes in the same manner found in interethnic interaction (Johnson, 1986). Johnson contends that social class position can be structurally viewed as a subcultural experience predicated on the verification of the individual's identity within a particular occupational and educational strata. Class levels operate as boundary mechanisms regulating family relationships, friendship networks, courting, recreational patterns, language usage, socio-economic security, power expectations, and opportunities. Options may vary radically at the extremes of class position and failure to recognize these factors in counseling can lead to distorted communication (Johnson, 1986).

Class is not synonymous with race, but in countries such as South Africa where racism resulted in widespread deprivation of opportunities for Blacks, issues of race and class have coincided with processes of oppression. Pinderhughes (1984) has documented the impact of power differences across ethnic and racial groups and reports significant variation in the feelings and behaviors of those who are "more powerful" and those who are "less powerful."

In a class-based analysis, Turton (1986) extends the notion of counselor encapsulation to the nature and functions of ideology, and to the material bases of individual experience, culture and ideology. For Turton, the ideology that encapsulates a counselor may have culture-specific elements, but attention might be more fruitfully directed towards those elements that reflect dominant social relations.

African working-class clients' lack of opportunities and perceived means of goal attainment have to be taken into account in counseling. Methods of counseling developed by and for members of the European and North American bourgeoisie are likely to be less effective when applied to problems experienced by working class Africans (Turton, 1986). South African counselors, typically drawn from the middle class, need to break out of traditional *modus operandi*, empathize with the hopes, fears, conflicts, and goals of the working class (Anonymous, 1986), and no longer be associated with "the privileged and powerful classes, with little understanding of the concerns and realities of the oppressed" (Berger & Lazarus, 1987, p. 13).

Bourgeois attitudes to working class patients may result in two subtle yet complex positions that could lead to working-class clients being denied therapy. The first subtle manifestation of bourgeois ideology may be expressed in the belief that adverse social conditions may give rise to personality disorder, which many professionals find difficult to dislodge (Hayes, 1986). Because of their chronicity and problematical course in treatment, personality-disordered patients have often been unpopular with clinicians (Lewis & Appleby, 1988; Paris, 1998). The view that members of the working class have a greater predisposition to personality-disorder is a deficit-oriented perspective.

The second subtle manifestation of bourgeois ideology may be the view that working-class problems are social problems, unamenable to therapy (Hayes, 1986). This position does the opposite of ignoring social realities; it exaggerates the social to the detriment of the individual requiring therapy. Some White therapists may feel that the lot of the working-class is so miserable that empathic counseling is likely to either be futile or to fuel feelings of misery unnecessarily. Thomas & Sillen (1972) state that:

Such awareness has led some psychiatrists to adopt a nihilistic attitude toward the treatment of poor Blacks. They contend that it is hopeless to treat a person who will continue to live in a pathogenic environment. Some even argue that the problems of a Black patient are so bound up with his oppression by the White power structure that he cannot be truly helped until racism has been wiped out. No matter what the goodwill of persons who take this position, they are in effect shutting the door of treatment facilities on patients with emotional problems or mental illness. The attitude appears militant, but is actually a counsel of exclusion. (p. 139)

Individualistically oriented practice runs the risk of infusing working class clients with bourgeois values, internalized from counselors via the therapy process (Turton, 1986). The counselor or therapist who operates unaware of larger system variables may be guilty of "symbolic violence" (Bourdieu & Passeron, 1977) through individual therapeutic interventions designed to help clients "feel better" about conditions beyond their control (Ivey, 1986, p. 288). Helping patients to adjust to oppressive conditions rather than to seek changes in those conditions is one reason why psychotherapy has sometimes been labeled as an opiate or instrument of oppression (Pinderhughes, 1973, p. 99) and psychology as "the handmaiden of the status quo" (Halleck, 1971). A number of progressive psychologists have baulked at mainstream psychology's claim to a value-free stance and at humanistic psychology's lack of a political agenda to address processes of socio-economic domination and oppression (e.g., Dawes, 1986; Seedat & Nell, 1992; Seedat, 1997; Turton, 1986; Vogelman, 1986).

There is a danger in adopting extreme positions with regard to the question of class and psychotherapy. Two extreme positions are identifiable (Richter et al., 1998): "the narrow professional with highly developed skills working in a circumscribed area and the generalist social agent required to implement and drive the social reform and development upon which the country has embarked" (p. 6). An overemphasis on either the social or the individual is likely to be problematic.

The empathy of counselors for working-class clients may be hindered by complex ideological factors. Moreover, interactions influenced by dominant social relations may be compounded in contexts, such as the South African one, where race and class have cohered because of racial discrimination.

RACE AND RACIAL IDENTITY

Race deserves a more central focus in counseling literature than it is usually afforded (Carter, 1995). For Carter "race organizes culture in the United States" (p. 44) and "is central to cultural groupings ... the superordinate locus of culture through which racial groups are identified" (p. 259). Carter contends that race is not just a cultural factor, but a psychological factor; race and racial identity—that is, an individual's level of psychological maturation associated with his or her racial group membership—are integral aspects of personality and human development.

Carter adheres to an interactional model (Helms, 1984) that understands racial identity to define the quality of therapeutic relationships, and which categorizes psychotherapeutic dyads according to similarities and dissimilarities in the racial identity states of participants. In a stage or levels model of racial identity, racial identity represents ego differentiation in the sense of self-definition or autonomy from other persons' points of view, and one's racial worldview may be evaluated as more or less mature depending on one's degree of liberation from racist perspectives. Less mature ego statuses derive definition from external sources, are simplistic, inaccurate, and unexamined group notions about race and race relations. More mature and differentiated racial identity ego statuses are internally derived through a personal process of exploration, discovery, integration, and maturation (Carter, 1995). Helms and Piper (1994) suggest that at any one point an individual has many levels of racial identity but only one dominant level. The predominant racial identity level operates psychologically as a worldview or ego state, and each level has its own constellation of emotions, beliefs, motives, and behaviors that influence its expression. Predominant racial identity levels operate psychologically as a worldview or ego state in psychotherapy as well, and client and counselor racial identity levels combine in therapy dyads to produce varied effects (Helms & Carter, 1991). Studies in the United States (Helms & Carter, 1991; Helms, 1990, 1994; Parham & Helms, 1985) reveal that the effects of racial identity on therapeutic processes vary depending on both the level of racial identity and the manner in which client and counselor racial identities combine.

Based on her research on how racial identity statuses interact in dyads, Helms (1984, 1990) has posited four relationship types: parallel, crossed, progressive, or regressive. In a parallel relationship, a client and a counselor of the same race are at similar levels of racial identity development, or the dyad's participants, although of different races, share similar attitudes about Blacks and Whites. In parallel relationships, racial issues are typically avoided with the intention of maintaining a pleasant, nonthreatening environment. Consequently, the dyad may be unable to deal with racial content even though the participants may have similar racial identity issues. The client and therapist operate as if they are color-blind, that is, as if there are no differences between members of different races and as if race is of no relevance, but their actions tend to be based on unspoken and subconscious assumptions about each other.

A progressive relationship occurs when the counselor's racial identity is at least one level more advanced than the client's is. In this type of relationship, counselors tend to perceive the counseling process as favorable when exploring clients' feelings, while clients are more content when support is provided or problematic behaviors are identified. When counselors focus on issues of race, clients may respond slowly and counselors may become upset, anxious, and angry. However, the therapeutic process may prove productive if the counselor can focus the client on treatment.

A regressive relationship exists when the client's racial identity status is at least one level more advanced than the counselor's is. In regressive dyads, counselors prefer to explore deep unconscious motivations and intrapsychic dynamics rather than current social realities. Counselors appear to be comfortable with racial issues only when they are discussed in terms of the client's dynamics and not the counselor's. In this relationship type, counselors may feel threatened by clients' better grasp of racial issues when compared to their own, while clients may be motivated to deal more directly with racial issues. The relationship dynamics may be characterized by conflict and the process may resemble a power struggle, with both participants having strong affective reactions to each other (Carter, 1995).

A crossed relationship involves participants of the same or different races, but whose racial identity statuses are opposite. In crossed dyads, counselors and clients both engage in educative strategies without empathizing with the other's racial attitudes. This may hinder therapeutic rapport and lead to early therapy termination.

No person or professional group is immune to the influence of racism, yet few training programs equip psychologists with adequate knowledge, attitudes, and skills for interracial work (Carter, p. 42). Well-intentioned therapists may be unaware that they are acting in inadvertently racist ways (Ridley, 1995). Therapists may not challenge their own behavior because of a lack of awareness of wrongdoing and an assumption that their good intentions automatically make them helpful (Pedersen, 1997, p. 31). However, the effectiveness of interventions rather than good intentions needs to be ascertained (Ridley, p. 10). Racism may be regarded as any practice which, intentional or not, excludes a racial or ethnic minority from enjoying the full rights, opportunities and responsibilities available to the majority population (Goldberg, 1994).

Social cognitions underlying social practices of oppression and exclusion are largely shaped through discursive communication within elite groups (Van Dijk, 1991). White psychologists comprise a particularly elite group for two reasons:

1. The White group has been historically advantaged, has had the power to control other groups, and has exercised that power; and
2. The power that accrues to those possessing recognized psychological knowledge is amplified by their legally and socially mandated interventions in matters pertaining to mental health.

The effects of oppression need not be deleterious to self-concept, but they can be. Race is an important aspect of one's identity and should be incorporated into models of personality development from which it has been absent (Carter, 1995). Racial identity has a bearing on personality development (Carter, 1995; Milner, 1997), yet few developmental theories address the impact of its influence.

The nature of their training does not equip mental health professionals to understand the impact of either race or racial identity on their clients' worldviews, interpersonal interactions, or therapy dynamics (Carter, 1995). Many mental health practitioners are personally and/or professionally unable to help their clients learn about, cope with, and grow in understanding concerning the influence of race in their personal and interpersonal lives. The way in which race is treated in mental health practice mirrors the way in which it is generally treated in society: race is a taboo topic, not valued and not discussed (Carter, pp. 267–268).

Ironically, one way in which psychologists may perpetuate racism is by adopting an attitude that was previously valued as reflecting true regard for Blacks; notably an attitude of color-blindness. Color-blindness in counseling is the tendency to deny a client's color and to try treating him or her like any other client. Griffith (1977) notes the following difficulties of a color-blind position:

1. Denying the color of the Black client disregards the central importance to that client of his or her Blackness, and ignores the impact of the therapist's Whiteness (Sager et al., 1972).
2. The Black client is likely to pick up the therapist's avoidance of the color issue. This reinforces barriers in the therapy relationship (Adams, 1970; Vontress, 1969).
3. Denying the impact of color and racism on the client's personality development abstracts the client from the social realities of his or her experiences.
4. Ignoring socio-cultural parameters of behavior associated with the Black client's behavior leads automatically to labeling deviations from White middle-class norms as pathological (Thomas & Sillen, 1972). The "illusion of color-blindness" (Adams, 1970; Cooper, 1973; Sabshin et al., 1970; Sager et al., 1972; Thomas & Sillen, 1972) contributes to the attitude that a Black client's culture is the same as that of the majority (dominant) culture (Griffith, p. 29).

Difficulties in problem conception, client assessment, and therapeutic rapport may lead to ineffective therapy where factors shaping racial identity are excluded from the therapy process (Carter, p. 23). At present, little consistent and reliable information is available on the topic of race and culture in therapy (Carter, p. 65). Much of what is known about race in psychotherapy "is grounded in a mixture of supposition, speculation, racism and personal bias" (Carter, p. 6).

Given the dearth of theories about race and identity development, the influence of race on individual and interpersonal interactions in a therapeutic setting and in society is unclear. Moreover, theoretical approaches to understanding race in psychotherapy have allowed mental health professionals to remain ignorant about themselves as members of a racial group and about how an individual incorporates race into identity (Carter, p. 83).

SUMMARY

White clinicians are likely to have distorted or inadequate knowledge of diverse client worldviews and therapy preferences. Their encapsulation may result in the rendering of inappropriate mental health services to the majority Black population, as well as to frequent misdiagnoses. Mental health practitioners need to educate themselves as to indigenous resources available for mental health and to consider how these mechanisms fit or clash with their professional training. An understanding of the mismatch between Western psychotherapies and local cultural perspectives, as well as their similarities, together with an appreciation of processes of acculturation, is required if counselors are to be liberated from a limitation of perspective.

It is, moreover, essential to the therapeutic endeavor for counselors to understand the impact of their racially informed attitudes and assumptions concerning clients in interracial contexts. Many counselors and therapists are ill equipped to deal with racially salient material. Professional training is generally inadequate on matters pertaining to race and racism, and therapists may be influenced by prevailing racist ideologies, unaware of how their racial prejudices translate into discriminatory work practices, and ignorant of the power of their own elite discourses.

Part II

Alternatives to Apartheid-Style Psychology

Human rights principles of equality and dignity provide a counterideology to racism and oppression. Despite the perturbing picture of apartheid-style elements in South African psychology and their resonance with international literature on racism and cultural insensitivity in counseling, there have been moves to democratize psychotherapy and psychological research. Links are made in the next two chapters between the human rights movement, the democratization of psychotherapy, and the ethos of postmodernism and social constructionism, which provide intellectual support for nonelitism and the limitation of mental health professionals' power. Theoretically, diverse literatures that share an antiauthoritarian commonality of perspective are drawn upon. Chapter 4 covers a wide range of material, beginning with human rights and democratic processes in both South Africa and the discipline of psychology. It is argued that there is considerable synchronicity between the ethical stance underlying human rights agendas and counseling practice. For example, both enshrine nondomination, egalitarianism, respect for the other in any encounter, and the tolerance of difference. Psychotherapeutic Relationships (Working, I-You, and Real) as well as systemic, community, and multicultural approaches are highlighted as reflective of antiauthoritarian concerns in psychotherapy. The discussion then moves in Chapter 5 to postmodern and constructionist perspectives that have an antihegemonic stance. These perspectives encourage researchers and therapists to critically reflect on their personal biases, countertransference issues, and contextual influences in psychotherapy.

4

Democratic and Client Empowering Initiatives

HUMAN RIGHTS

"Human rights" is commonly taken to refer to rights that every human being is entitled to and to have protected (Reoch, 1994). The ideology underpinning human rights reflects profound human aspirations that have their antecedents in the world's great religions and cultures (Sieghart, 1988). For instance, many religions which recognize the Divine creation of humankind give impetus to the applicability of human rights as independent of any merit or guilt, on the argument that being human, *imago Dei*, warrants full entitlement to seek rights (Harris, 1997). The principle of equality and human dignity finds consensus among many people of various backgrounds (Pagels, 1979).

The first *explicit* recognition that every human being has rights that are to be recognized, as opposed to conferred by society, emerged during the Enlightenment (Adams, 1997; Pagels, 1979). The theory of human rights as "inalienable" was articulated at the time of the Civil War in England, during the framing of the United States Constitution, and during the French Revolution, fought in the name of "liberty, equality and fraternity" (Pagels, p. 6). In the wake of indignation at atrocities perpetrated during World War II, the notion of human rights was codified in international law (Sieghart, 1988, p. 2). The Universal Declaration of Human Rights was largely formulated to provide a counter-ideology to the racist and fascist ideologies of Nazism (Shivji, 1999), and the political philosophy of human rights has since taken root and manifested itself in diverse international treaties and declarations (Buergenthal, 1979; Devenish, 1998; Keightley, 1992).

In South Africa, the diverse political traditions and perspectives that informed the struggle against apartheid shared convergent perspectives that insisted on human rights. Contemporary South African political culture might be said to be rooted in the distinctive perspectives of Christian humanism; the Gandhian tradition of nonviolent resistance to oppression (satyagraha); and the African "ubuntu" principle (Nagan & Atkins, 2002). The concept of ubuntu literally means that *people are people through people*, and stresses the principle of reciprocally honoring the inherent worth of all members of the community. The merger of a version of socialist humanism with European roots and an African version of socialist humanism implicit in the ubuntu idea, reveals core principles of democratic entitlement, respect for civil and political rights, cultural and economic equity, and cultural, gender-based and racial justice. These perspectives on human rights gave the struggle against injustice in South Africa a high moral and ethical basis (Nagan & Atkins, 2002).

The Doctrine of Due Process

Human rights may be substantive or procedural (van der Vyfer, 1976). Substantive rights include personal rights (such as the right to life, liberty, and property); civil rights; political rights; economic rights; cultural rights and social rights (such as freedom of association, and freedom to marry and have a family) (Carpenter, 1987, p. 94). Mentally ill people are frequently denied some or all of these substantive rights.

Procedural rights relate to the administration of justice and the "due process of law." Due process presumes that a person should be free, and requires that rigid procedures be followed before an individual's liberty is removed (Packer, 1964). The involuntary confinement of mentally ill patients has largely ignored the human rights doctrine of due process. As elsewhere, in South Africa, due process elements were rendered vacuous by judicial officers' limited knowledge of mental illness, their assumption that treatment cannot hurt, and deference to medical opinion without legal safeguards (Haysom, Strous & Vogelman, 1990; Korenberg & Korenberg, 1981).

A due process approach may be compared favorably for the protection of the human rights of mentally ill persons against a social control approach to mental illness. The efficient processing of patients as rapidly as possible so that there is enough space for new patients entering the public health system, which occurs in order to contain health care costs (Eisenberg, 1995; Swartz, 1998), is more conducive to social control than a culture of human rights. Psychiatry has been accused of "getting rid" of patients while appearing to care (L. Swartz, 1991). An appeal for the increased appreciation of due process rights of the mentally ill has been made by Haysom, Strous and Vogelman (1990) within a discourse on human rights. These authors recommended an amendment to procedures for patient confinement contained in the Mental Health Act, the judicial inspection of psychiatric facilities, the abolition of secrecy, and greater transparency in the study of psychiatric facilities.

The Right to Equality in Health Care

From a human rights perspective, the limitation of professional time in diagnosis and treatment, in order to improve cost-efficiency ratios, is insidious given the inferior treatment of disempowered groups within mental health systems. Racism may directly advantage dominant White society by excluding Black staff from managerial posts and through easing out Black patients from time-consuming treatment modalities (Fernando, 1988). Ridley (1995) reports that disempowered clients tend to be misdiagnosed more frequently than warranted, and usually receive more severe diagnoses than privileged, usually White clients. They tend to be assigned junior and less trained staff and frequently receive low-cost treatment consisting of minimal contact, medicine only, or custodial care rather than intensive psychotherapy. They show a higher rate of premature termination and dropout from therapy, and are confined to longer inpatient care. They are underrepresented in private treatment facilities, overrepresented in public treatment facilities, and report more dissatisfaction and unfavorable impressions regarding treatment. In the United States, Black patients are more frequently diagnosed psychotic, involuntarily hospitalized and given powerful antipsychotic drugs, than are their White counterparts (Cole & Pilisuk, 1976; Littlewood & Lipsedge, 1997, p. 55; Willie, Kramer & Brown, 1973). In Britain, poor understanding of social determinants of mental illness and psychiatric practices, inadequate investigation into patients' perspective and resources, greater emphasis on hospital as opposed to community issues, avoidance of racism issues, and little liaising between minority group members and service providers, contribute to concerns that there are inequalities in health care services (Littlewood & Lipsedge, p. vii). There are few psychotherapists committed to working with ethnic minorities, and minorities are less likely to receive individual or group therapy (Littlewood & Lipsedge, p. vii).

The human rights approach takes issue with such inequalities in the provision of mental health services. An influx in publications addressing health as a human rights issue over the course of the last few years underlies concerns as to: "the potential abuse of advanced technologies, the scarcity of resources to meet essential health care needs, discrimination against people with impaired health and the unequal distribution of health care consumption both between and within countries" (Hendriks & Toebes, 1998, pp. 322–323).

Discrimination by a state among its inhabitants in the matter of access to limited resources, such as doctors, is unlawful in international human rights law (Sieghart, 1988, p. 10). The concept of nondiscrimination is fundamental to all theories of human rights (Sieghart, 1988) and the right to health is firmly embedded in international human rights law (Hendriks & Toebes, 1998).

The mental health system has often, wittingly or unwittingly, stereotyped Blacks negatively and stigmatized the mentally ill. Blacks and the mentally ill have in common that they have frequently been alienated, isolated from mainstream society, and deprived of their human rights. Human rights provisions that focus on inclusionary group participation, equality, and nondiscrimination, offer a contraposition to these exclusionary mental health practices.

Nonauthoritarianism

In South Africa, concerns relating to the assumed pathogenic nature of institutionalized racism, human rights violations in the provision of mental health services, and possible abuses of psychiatry under the apartheid system, emerged at the same time that a related human rights debate was happening in the West. This debate centered on accusations of a Soviet propensity to label political dissenters as insane in violation of their intrinsic rights. International concern that mental health professionals can easily abuse their professional standing was sparked off by allegations of Soviet misuses of psychiatry as a penal tool (Cohen, 1989; Fireside, 1979). At the same time that the Soviet psychiatry dispute was unfolding, the antipsychiatry movement criticized mental health practices in the West as placing too much power in the hands of a few mental health professionals.

Agitated by what they perceived to be psychiatry's monopolistic hold over the mental health arena, the antipsychiatry movement viewed the development of techniques for behavioral control to represent a threat to individual human rights. Thomas Szasz (1970) criticized Western psychiatric practice on the basis that it sought to control behavior which deviates from a psychological norm by labeling it as mental illness, while Goffmann (1968) contested the ability of mental institutions to provide therapeutic benefits for their patients, and suggested that mental institutions damage inmates by reducing their sense of self worth, stripping them of autonomy and stigmatizing them as mentally incompetent. Although the antipsychiatry movement took issue with the mainstream psychiatric establishment in the United States, their view that psychiatry was susceptible to authoritarian manipulation appeared to be corroborated by revelations of dissident internment in the Soviet Union.

There were ideological points of contact between the discourse on human rights around Soviet psychiatry, the antipsychiatry movement, and accusations of complicity by mental health professionals in South Africa in instances of state-sponsored terrorism, such as torture, and the maintenance of inferior standards of mental health care for the disenfranchized majority. The need for limitations to be placed on the power of mental health professionals that was made both locally and internationally reflected support for an ideology of equality and the rights of those labeled mentally ill.

From a standpoint of suspicion of psychiatry as a tool for social control, the Fourth Annual North American Conference on Human Rights and Psychiatric Oppression held in Boston in May 1976 adopted the following resolution (Horowitz, 1982):

We reject compulsory commitments to mental hospitals. We reject the mental health care system, because it is by nature despotic and acts as an extra-legal police force for the suppression of cultural and political dissidents. We reject the concept of mental illness because it is used to justify involuntary commitment, and in particular we reject the imprisonment of people who have committed no crime....We reject the use of psychiatric terminology, because it is intrinsically stigmatizing and degrading, nonscientific and magical. (p. 251)

Laissez-faire contentions that the less mental health services that are provided the better, may emanate out of antipsychiatry arguments. Such a radical perspective would ignore the possible benefits of mental health care (Vogelman, 1986). The antipsychiatry movements' concerns have, however, dovetailed with human rights concerns that attitudes concerning mental health are often influenced by both social and political constructs, that there exists a danger of mental health being used at the cost of individual human rights to subjugate challenges to the social order, and that there is a need for checks and balances to avoid the potential abuse of power by mental health professionals. Compatible with these concerns, the postmodernist movement has generated renewed calls for an exploration of moral-political projects that are embedded in a sense of justice (Derrida, 1983) rather than in given diagnoses and descriptions of pathology, which have potential to oppress people as they pretend to help them (Parker, 1999, p. 2).

Cultural Diversity and Equality

Cultural diversity, equality, and nondiscrimination are recursive themes in current debates and international standard setting on the protection of group rights (Strydom, 1998).

The core value of this principle (equality) is that all people have equal worth. When the legal order that both shapes and mirrors our society treats some people as outsiders as though they were worth less than others, those people have been denied equal protection. Mediated by the antisubjugation principle the equal protection clause asks whether the particular conditions complained of, examined in their social and historical context, are a manifestation or a legacy of official oppression. (Tribe, cited in Devenish, 1998, p. 48)

The notion of equality, central to human rights ideology, refers to equality in law rather than to human sameness (Kentridge, 1996; Sieghart, 1988). Human rights law does not treat individuals as equal but as different from each other to the extent that they are unique and entitled to equal rights (Sieghart, 1988). In the words of the 1789 French Declaration of the Rights of Man and the Citizen, people are "free and equal in *respect of rights*" (Sieghart, 1988, p. 10). A fundamental concept has been the prevention of forced assimilation. Minority groups are recognized as having concurrently the right to full equality with the majority and preservation of separate identities (Dinstein, 1976).

The concept of cultural diversity and equality as a basic human right finds expression in the postapartheid South African Constitution, which provides that:

The State may not unfairly discriminate directly or indirectly against anyone on one or more grounds, including race, gender, sex, pregnancy, marital status, ethnic or social origin, color, sexual orientation, age, disability, religion, conscience, belief, culture, language and birth. (Chapter 2 art 9[3]). Persons belonging to a cultural, religious or linguistic community may not be denied the right with other members of that community—to enjoy their culture, practice their religion and use their language; and to form, join and maintain cultural, religious and linguistic associations and other organs of civil society. (Chapter 2 art 31[1], cited by Nortier & Theron, 1998, p. 230)

The theme of equality in diversity, when translated to the mental health field, imposes special obligations on counselors. Culturally encapsulated therapists may unintentionally contribute to cultural oppression because of their ignorance of cultural norms of diverse client groups (Hickson, Christie, & Shmukler, 1990; Hickson & Kriegler, 1996). Counselor encapsulation may negatively affect therapeutic rapport, transference–countertransference phenomena and racial identity interactions. In fact, cultural misunderstandings, intolerance, and racist preconceptions may distort psychological treatment at every stage of the process; for example, patient acceptance, the availability of facilities, the nature of therapeutic relationships, goal setting with clients, and the evaluation of therapy outcomes (Thomas & Sillen, 1972, p. 135).

Psychotherapy in interracial and multicultural contexts is often hindered by cultural, class, and language differences between counselors and clients (Sue & Sue, 1977). The importation of a human rights culture into mental health could help to conscientize practitioners to the need for multicultural awareness, skills, and knowledge in order to avoid cultural subjugation. The notion of self-determination as a composite cultural right has the advantage of taking on board discourses on participatory democracy, accountability, and consultative participation at "people's" level in the continuous process of decision making. These themes, which are of concern to human rights activists (Shivji, p. 270), also find expression in the democratization of psychological practice.

MOVES TO DEMOCRATIZATION

The new protection and advancement of human dignity in South African legislation, which aspires to international human rights standards, is contemporaneous to moves toward the democratization of psychology. A limitation of executive power, which characterizes the human rights approach to democracy, finds expression in the mental health field in concerns to limit professional authoritarianism and elitism.

In the political arena, the limitation of power is designed to facilitate government by persuasion rather than coercion (Mureinik, 1994). A culture of obedience to authority, characteristic of oppression, is replaced by a culture of justification (Mureinik, 1994): "a culture in which every exercise of power is expected to be justified, in which the leadership given by government rests on the cogency of the case offered in defence of its decisions, not the fear inspired by the force at its command" (p. 32).

South Africa has turned its back on its apartheid past and has moved away from nonparticipation in international and regional human rights conventions (Dlamini, 1997; Dugard, 1998). The 1996 Constitution of the RSA was adopted "to establish a society based on democratic values, social justice and fundamental human rights" (Malherbe & Rautenbach, 1996, preface). The bill of rights contained in chapter two of the South African Constitution enshrines democratic values of human dignity, equality, and freedom (Dlamini, 1997). It is one of the most comprehensive and far-reaching bills of rights in the world. South Africa has been transformed into one of the most advanced societies as far as the statutory protection and advancement of human rights is concerned (de Groof & Malherbe, 1997).

Psychologists socialized in apartheid South Africa have experienced the country's ideological transition to democracy. They have also been exposed to attempts to democratize psychotherapy. The limitation of unchecked powers as a human rights theme is mirrored in the mental health arena in concerns to limit injudicious power practices by professionals.

The implication of professional codes of conduct as a device for protecting and aiding the public implies a recognition that within the field of mental health psychologists have the power to inflict harm, and restraints are needed to limit this power (L. Swartz, 1988). Excesses or abuses of power may inhere in "knowing" what is best for clients, minimizing clients' autonomy by excluding them from decision-making processes, stigmatizing individuals with deficit-oriented labels, and neglecting to consider social injustices in nonintrapsychic terms (Prilleltensky, 1997).

The new Ethical Code of Professional Conduct of The Professional Board for Psychology in South Africa (2002) states that:

Psychologists shall respect the constitutional right of all to dignity and the right to have that dignity respected and protected and not to be discriminated against unfairly on any grounds....Psychologists shall respect the dignity and worth of the individual and shall strive for the preservation and protection of fundamental human rights in all professional conduct....Psychologists shall respect the right of others to hold values, attitudes, beliefs, and opinions that differ from their own...shall not impose on clients, employees, research participants, students, supervisees, trainees, or others over whom psychologists have or had authority any stereotypes of behavior, values or roles related to age, belief, birth, conscience, colour, culture, disability, disease, ethnic and social origin, gender, language, marital status, pregnancy, race, religion, sexual orientation, socio-economic status, or any basis proscribed by law...shall not engage in unfair discrimination (and) shall make every effort to ensure that language-appropriate and culture-appropriate services are made available to clients. (Section 2)

Concerns that the rights of mental health service recipients should be protected are also reflected in South Africa's first new draft law on mental health care in 29 years. The new Mental Health Care Bill provides, for example, for more regular reviews of patients in involuntary care to assess their suitability for discharge, and sets up review boards to do this. It defines how basic human rights are to be interpreted in relation to individuals unable to exercise independent judgment. It further provides that individuals subject to involuntary institutional care are entitled to legal representation and stipulates that they should be eligible for legal aid if they cannot afford a lawyer. It also lifts the blanket of secrecy that the old Mental Health Act threw over psychiatric hospitals by virtually banning media access (*The Star* 26 September 2001).

In addition to formal regulations that stipulate the protection of human rights in mental health, a large number of schools of psychology emphasize the importance of freedom of choice for clients. The democratization of psychotherapy represents a move away from nonconsensual manipulation of clients and implies collaboration between therapists and clients in a shared process of mutual consultation. Coercive practices and excessive reliance on the expert professional as an authority figure to effect behavioral change are anathema to a human rights ideology of democratization. Democracy presupposes a world in which one acts *with* people rather than on their behalf (Louw, 1983).

The Working Alliance, the I–You Relationship, the Real Relationship, and systemic approaches are all modalities that have tackled the need to place limitations on the professional authority of counselors. Community psychologists and the multicultural counseling movement have also addressed the need to make psychology more accountable to its users. These approaches are now discussed in turn.

THE WORKING ALLIANCE/RELATIONSHIP

The aim of the Working Alliance is a therapeutic relationship philosophy designed to explicitly involve clients in consensual engagement. For many schools of psychotherapy, the Working Alliance is crucial and necessary for effective therapy (Clarkson, 1990). It stresses partnership between the client and counselor and underscores the responsibility of the client in the therapeutic endeavor (Egan, 1986, p. 137).

The establishment of a Working Relationship is a complex issue in interracial therapy in South Africa. Joining with clients in a democratically participative manner should influence the therapist's praxis and therapeutic program (Seedat & Nell, 1990). South African therapists, who are typically White, need to join emotionally with clients who have been hurt by White people; otherwise, the authority of the therapist and the submission of a client can replicate broader social processes of power, control, and oppression. Western-style therapy may sometimes fail by unwittingly perpetuating social power structures, and imposing solutions that have not been explored and negotiated with clients, thereby reactivating their existential pain.

A number of writers have commented on the difficulty of achieving mutually accepting relationships between Black clients and White therapists because of cultural differences and ingrained attitudes (Griffith, 1977; Jackson, 1973; Vontress, 1969). White therapists may have beliefs of questionable validity, gathered from the professional literature, the attitudes of training supervisors, and their own conscious and unconscious feelings and attitudes about Black people, which interfere with the establishment of therapeutic rapport (Greene, 1985). Black clients may express subtle or overt hostility toward White therapists, based on misgivings concerning White racism. These factors threaten the Working Alliance.

Common therapy factors which seem to foster the Working Alliance and which could be of particularly beneficial import in interracial settings are the setting of mutually accepted goals, coupled with therapist attributes of accurate empathy, positive regard for the client, nonpossessive warmth, and congruence or genuineness (Truax & Mitchell, 1971). These positive therapist attributes facilitate the development of trust, client openness and self-disclosure (Egan 1986; Truax & Carkhuff, 1965). They are attributes emphasized by humanistic psychologists in particular, although "virtually all schools of psychotherapy accept the notion that these or related therapist relationship variables are important for significant progress in psychotherapy" (Lambley, cited by Clarkson, 1990, p.150). According to Pedersen (1997), effective counselors vary the power of therapeutic interventions according to a client's changing needs; in some instances exerting more power through interpretation and confrontation, and sometimes exerting less power through reflection or nondirective accommodation, in order to negotiate a successful Working Alliance/coalition relationship between clients and counselors.

A contradiction in having clients blindly follow therapist dictates is that, however well intentioned the therapist may be, the client becomes overly dependent on the therapist, contrary to therapeutic goals of fostering client autonomy (Jones & Seagull, 1977). Therapists committed to the optimization of client freedom need to be sensitive to their clients' needs rather than work within rigid frameworks and impose their own goals. Encouraging clients to set mutually agreed upon goals in a collaborative manner (Ridley, 1995) and the rendering of genuine empathy and positive regard for clients are compatible with the human rights focus on dignity, and are dimensions of the Working Alliance that contradict a culture of authority.

THE I–YOU RELATIONSHIP

The I–You relationship represents one of the most democratic devolutions of expertise in psychotherapy. According to Martin Buber (1970) there are two ways of relating: I–You relationships or I–It relationships. The I–You relationship is one of intimacy, mutuality, sharing, and trust. The I–It relationship refers to the way that a person relates to a reified object and is devoid of mutuality or respect. To relate to a person as an impersonal "it" positions that person as a thing to be possessed, used and exploited rather than as an individual who can be appreciated in dialogical interaction. The I–You relationship underpins many strands of existential psychology and, through engaging with clients as equals in direct relationship, aims to counter the subjugation of human dignity inherent in I-It relationships.

The I–You therapeutic relationship is an existential encounter where the therapist and client reveal themselves to each other stripped of their usual defenses. When the therapist judges it appropriate and timely to trust or delight the patient with a sense of shared personhood (Clarkson, 1990), he or she may make self-disclosures, provided that this serves to meet the client's needs rather than to gratify the therapist's own needs.

The I–You relationship contradicts the manner in which many clients with self-pathologies relate to others, such as their therapists, as part-objects which are not valued for any qualities beyond their abilities to soothe or esteem the client's fragile sense of self (Kohut, 1977). It also contradicts therapeutic interventions in which clients are treated like things by therapists. In his "le syndrome du Bon Dieu," Strauss (1981, cited in *Living*, 1988) voices concern that omnipotent-feeling doctors, through a display of bio-medical knowledge and technical skills, frequently treat patients as if they were objects, rather than equal partners in a decision-making process aimed at better health. When clients are related to as dehumanized "its" they become disavowed of their "you" contributions to dialogical interaction and they become subservient to "expert opinion."

Positivist understandings of psychology as a value free science may lead to a perspective that clients are passive pawns to be acted upon. For positivists there appears to be consensus in society concerning reality and norms and an elite capable of understanding the "true nature" of behavior. The consensus defines behavior as either normal or deviant, the elite determines rules, and it is the therapist's task to provide efficient treatment of deviant behavior (Young, 1981). When therapists set themselves up as experts, clients' phenomenological understandings and dialogical contributions may be minimized. The I–You Relationship contests such processes by emphasizing equality and nonauthoritarianism in the counselor–client relationship, for the protection and advancement of human dignity and self-esteem.

REAL RELATIONSHIP

The Real Relationship—also called the basic human relationship (Egan, 1986) or Core Relationship—which is emphasized in person-centered or client-centered therapies, shares with dialogical I–You approaches a repudiation of positivist notions. Both the Real Relationship and the I–You relationship challenge the role of the therapist as an expert investigator, diagnostician and interpreter. Client-centered approaches place greater faith in clients' capacities for self-direction than in therapeutic interpretation. It is the goal of client-centered therapy to provide a nondirective, safe climate conducive to clients' self-exploration, so that clients can recognize blocks to growth and experience aspects of self that were formerly denied or distorted.

The Real Relationship is the human base on which the helping alliance is built and is characterized by the openness and genuineness of both the client and the counselor (Egan, 1986, p. 138). Attending, listening, empathy, challenge, respect, and genuineness are all facets of the Real Relationship.

Client-centered approaches share allegiance to the phenomenological method where client verbalizations are accepted in their essence and are not interrogated for deep underlying meanings. A specific advantage of working within the Real Relationship in interracial contexts is the potential facilitation of a comfortable and unconstrained relationship of mutual trust and confidence. The therapist facilitates rapport in the Real Relationship by suspending critical judgment. Adopting a stance of "unconditional positive regard," the therapist communicates a deep and genuine caring for the client as a person with potentialities, in a manner uncontaminated by evaluation (Rogers, 1967). This contradicts negatively evaluative positions where therapists neither see nor treat an individual (Kagan, 1964) but make generalizations, such as racially stereotyped assumptions, which "lead to categorical prescriptions and the attendant loss of the client's uniqueness and worth" (Calia, cited by Jones & Seagull, 1977, p. 851). An ideographic approach to counseling (Ridley, 1995, pp. 81–105) acknowledges the uniqueness of each individual, and that each client should be understood from his or her unique frame of reference (Rogers, 1961) rather than as a group representative.

Client-centered approaches that are characterized by the fostering of the Real Relationship may permit greater client autonomy, rapport building, and emotional joining because of their nonjudgmental phenomenological underpinnings. However, criticisms have been leveled at client-centered approaches as fetishizing human subjectivity and ignoring processes of socio-economic domination and oppression (Cloete & Pillay, 1988; Dawes, 1986; Ivey, 1986; Seedat & Nell, 1992; Turton, 1986; Vogelman, 1986). Client-centered therapy may nevertheless be credited as the first attempt to democratize therapy (Heather, 1976, p. 128). Properly contextualised, the humanistic approach underpinning the Real Relationship can have value if used as the basis for self-awareness, and the exploration of such issues as the impact of self-estrangement and victimization on human relationships (Hickson & Kriegler, 1996, p. 24). Opportunities for self-exploration and self-realization, which characterize the Real Relationship, are fundamental tenets of democratic practice.

SYSTEMIC FAMILY THERAPY

Nonauthoritarianism and democratic ideals underpin recent trends in family therapy. Systemic family therapy recognized that emotional problems experienced by a family member are not that family member's problem alone but represent dysfunction within a family system. Concern that therapists may abuse their power by pathologizing families, as the family had pathologized its index patient, has led to the development of "critical" family therapy (Parker, 1999, p. 6).

Systemic family therapies that follow a critical approach are increasingly being influenced by "Fourth Wave Therapies" (O'Hanlon, 1992). Influenced by postmodernism, social constructionism and second order cybernetics (Maturana, 1978), the Fourth Wave movement views the possession of psychological "truths" by experts as a myth. The movement focuses on the democratization of psychological knowledge so as to overcome power inequalities inherent in colonial attitudes to psychotherapy (Barry & Guilfoyle, 1998). Influenced by Maturana's conception of unilinear attempts to specify another person's thoughts and to direct people unilaterally as "violence," the movement veers away from the notion of therapists as experts who can see into and inform another person of his or her "true self." The focus is on dialogical therapist–client cooperation and coevolvement.

According to proponents of a paradigm of evolutionary systemic change, therapists need to guard against imposing their beliefs, attitudes and assumptions on clients from diverse backgrounds (Dell, 1982, 1985; De Shazer, 1982, 1984; Luckhurst, 1985; Powis, 1989; Prigogine, 1978). In family therapy a context of neutral observation can be created if a therapist takes time to check out family perceptions, stays as close as possible to the family's worldview, and provides a context in which the family can "research themselves" (Powis, 1988). When the therapist acts as a change-agent rather than as a context-creator, the family may lose its freedom to mobilize creatively to deal with the problem at hand (Parry, 1984). The therapist should therefore ask, "How can I stop becoming a chronic therapist to this family?" (Boscolo, Cecchin, Campbell, & Draper, 1985). Therapists do not make changes in families (Penn, 1982), they merely provide the context in which the family structure is transformed according to its own singular laws (Elkaim, 1981; Hoffman, 1981). Mental health practitioners, according to this philosophy, need "to abandon the idea of the therapist as a bullfighter, pushing and pulling the family to where he wanted it" (Hoffman, 1981, p. 347). The call has been: "for a description of family therapy that is not based on a conflict model but rather is based on a cooperative effort between the component subsystems of therapist and family by removing the artificial barrier between the therapist subsystem and the family subsystem" (De Shazer, 1982, p. 82).

Recent trends in family therapy that embrace the democratic ideal of self-realization and nonauthoritarianism attempt to limit intentional and unintentional abuses of professional power. They represent determined commitment to the democratization of psychotherapy.

COMMUNITY PSYCHOLOGY

The field of community psychology is reflective of a diverse range of ideas. Concerns that run through the field of community psychology are that social problems affect personal functioning and that services to deal with life difficulties must be equitable and appropriate (Bender, 1976; Heller & Monahan, 1977; Rappaport, 1977). Community psychology identifies the need to democratize service delivery with reference to psychotherapy's sidestepping of the poor. Shortages of accessible mental health services and expensive treatments that are insensitive to the economic plight and political disempowerment of the "have-nots" are identified as reasons to democratize psychotherapeutic endeavors.

Psychology may be considered as essentially an elitist service, presently meeting the needs of only a small, privileged sector of society. To address the mental health needs of the Black majority in South Africa, a community psychology approach states that the primary area of focus should be on pertinent social problems. Community psychology has moved toward the provision of alternative services in an attempt to make the fields of applied psychology more effective in the delivery of services and more responsible to the needs of the community (Bender, 1976). The major values and aims of community psychology include empowerment and competency, prevention, an ecological perspective, socially useful research, an appreciation of cultural relativity and diversity, community and organizational development, and social advocacy (Heller & Monahan, 1977; Ivey, 1986; Rappaport, 1977).

While a community mental health model encourages communities and their members to develop better coping strategies and strengths so as to reduce the negative impact which the social environment has on individuals, the community social action model stresses that the causes of social problems are located within the structural arrangements of society. Arguing that mental health is difficult to ensure in a community in the context of repression and domination, the model encourages the mobilization and organization of powerless social groups, with a view to shifting the power balance and instituting broader structural changes (Seedat, 1998, p. 43).

The social action model encourages attempts to increase community morale, tap community resources, develop social skills, and generate opportunities for promoting local leadership. By strengthening communities and community leadership at a grass-roots level, it is intended to weaken the iniquitous centralization of authority that is located beyond the reach of ordinary community members. The role of the community psychologist in the social action model is of a community mobilizer cum conscientizer (Seedat, p. 45).

The community mental health model, which aims to facilitate the development of community members' coping strategies and strengths in reaction to negative social forces, raises the question whether concessions are not made to the prevailing social order by effecting an adjustment to it through relieving symptoms (Bulhan, 1985). According to Rappaport (1981), the potential for this to occur may be counteracted by the concept of "empowerment." The concept of empowerment is particularly important for groups that have learnt to see themselves as helpless or as having few options (Mulvey, 1988). It is a construct that links individual strengths, natural helping systems and proactive behaviors to matters of social policy and change whereby individuals gain psychological mastery or control over their lives in democratic participation in the life of a community (Rappaport, 1987). The implications of the approach revolve around its ethos of politically explicit personal and collective power and its emphasis on rights, entitlements, and nondomination (Prilleltensky, 1997). Empowerment-oriented approaches engage professionals as collaborators instead of as authoritative experts, in the exploration of environmental influences on social problems and the enhancement of self-determination (Perkins & Zimmerman, 1995).

MULTICULTURAL COUNSELING

The inclusion of disempowered social groups as recipients of mental health services is a fundamental concern for the multicultural counseling movement. Multicultural counseling literature suggests that culturally diverse clients might avoid dominant culture mental health services to prevent the erosion of their own values and cultural identity where those services might in fact increase acculturative stress among consumers (Pedersen, 1982). Multicultural counseling recognizes that clients and counselors have to work through and beyond their cultural differences. The multicultural perspective seeks to provide a conceptual framework that recognizes pluralistic diversity while at the same time suggesting bridges of shared concern that bind culturally different persons to one another (Sue, Ivey, & Pedersen, 1996). Counselors are encouraged to view themselves as a product of their own upbringing, to move beyond the confines of cultural encapsulation, and to be flexible with diverse client groups. The multicultural movement recognizes that the authentic counselor: "regardless of the worldview identification, possesses a wholesome appreciation for both his or her values and those of the client. This authenticity allows the counselor to be personally and objectively involved in the counseling process without threatening the client's freedom, rights and integrity" (Smith, cited by Hickson & Kriegler, 1996, p. 23).

Pedersen's multicultural view is that if we consider age, life-style, socio-economic status, and sex-role differences in addition to ethnic and nationality differences, there is a multicultural dimension in every counseling relationship. Because culture is within the person, developing multicultural awareness, skill, and knowledge becomes both an opportunity and obligation for the professional counselor (Pedersen, 1988). Pedersen (1999) asserts multiculturalism as an inclusive paradigm, a "fourth force" that compliments the three forces of behaviorism, humanism, and the psychodynamic approach by contextualizing the discipline of psychology within a culture-centered dimension.

According to Pedersen (2000), thousands of different culturally learned social roles compete, complement, and cooperate with one another in each person. A multicultural identity is *complex* (incorporating a great many cultures at the same time) and *dynamic* (in that only a few cultures are salient at any one point in time). Only when behavior is understood within a context of a person's salient social system variables of ethnographic, demographic, status, and affiliation variables—as they influence values and expectations—will the meaning of that person's behavior become clear.

Hickson and Kriegler (1996) outline the following issues that have been of concern to multicultural researchers:

1. Racial differences in the therapy encounter can impede therapeutic rapport (Vontress, 1969, 1979).
2. Language barriers, class-bound values, and culture-bound values threaten the counseling relationship (Padilla, Ruiz & Alvarez, 1975).
3. Racial and ethnic factors may result not only in diminished trust and rapport but also in the under utilization of mental health services, or in premature client termination (Sue & Sue, 1977).
4. Suggestions for appropriate cross-cultural counseling have been criticized for depicting stereotypes and caricatures. Cultural sensitivity requires counselors to adopt an accommodating attitude to members of different cultural groups and to avoid comparing cultures as "better" or "worse" than each other (Ahia, 1984).
5. The counseling of persons of culturally diverse backgrounds by persons not trained or competent to work with such groups has been recognized by the American Psychological Association as unethical (Korman, 1974).
6. Similarities and differences in clients of diverse cultures need to be recognized, appreciated, and respected.

The multicultural perspective contends that all cultures are coequal in the sense that there are many and different ways of being human (Hickson & Kriegler, 1996, p. 8). Pedersen (1988, 1991) has emphasized the term "multiculturalism" as a move away from exotic perspectives of culture in which certain groups are implicated as superior to others. Multiculturalism thus serves as a counter-ideology to unicultural parochialism:

Culture is the only construct in the social sciences that makes it possible for two people to disagree—in their behaviors, for example—without one necessarily being right and the other wrong when they are from different cultures. Multicultural awareness makes it possible to value both the ways we are similar *and* the ways we are different. The similarities of common-ground expectations for trust, respect, fairness and success require the cooperation of people who have attached different, and sometimes conflicting, behaviors to those shared expectations. (Pedersen cited in Hickson & Kriegler, 1996)

The following characteristics of cross-cultural or multicultural training models may be identified (Hickson & Kriegler, 1996):

1. An assumption that ethnic or cultural background influences worldview and how a person understands life and its problems.
2. An emphasis on learning about various cultural groups and worldviews in order to better understand how an individual from a particular group may experience life and its problems.
3. A focus on teaching counseling skills and interventions appropriate for use with members of various ethnic groups. (pp. 11–12)

A factor that mitigates against effective multicultural counseling may be the therapist's socialization in a racist and ethnocentric society (Bloombaum, Yamamoto, & James, 1968; Casas, 1984; Vontress, 1981). Moreover, the advancement of multicultural counseling sometimes requires "superflexibility" on the part of counselors, "elastic modifications" of sound principles (Wohl, 1981), and the abandonment of traditional theory and technique, sometimes by students who have not yet acquired them (Pedersen, 1988). Multicultural training, states Pedersen (1988), "is far from a precise science, but it continues to build on the hope that past mistakes need not be repeated and the knowledge that failure of multicultural contact is almost always enormously expensive and often tragic" (pp. 21–22). Pedersen recommends that training for increased multicultural understanding should generate experience-based learning about one's self in an active role, with the correct balance of safety and challenge to facilitate counselor growth.

Multicultural awareness, knowledge and skills have been recognized as basic competencies for multicultural counseling (Hickson & Kriegler, 1996; Pedersen, 1988, 1997; Pedersen & Ivey, 1993; Sue, Arrendondo, & McDavis, 1992). Awareness means being aware of personal prejudices and biases and moving towards the goal of valuing and respecting differences. Multicultural counselors should ideally apply a pluralistic philosophy and refrain not only from the imposition of culturally dominant beliefs, but from attitudes of paternalism and condescension as well (Hickson & Kriegler, p. 145). Cultural knowledge refers to the acquisition of information regarding one's own and other cultural values, worldviews, and social norms. Skills refer to the ability to accurately and appropriately receive and send both verbal and nonverbal messages. Counselors in multiracial settings must be open and flexible enough to change their approach in order to meet the needs of diverse client groups (Hickson & Kriegler, pp. 145–147).

The multicultural perspective's pertinence to the South African context is that it recognizes both pluralistic diversity as well as common concerns of people from different cultural groups (Hickson & Kriegler, 1996). The rehabilitation of multicultural psychology as an essential basis for an egalitarian psychology (Nell, 1993) would be apposite to the recognition that for psychologists cultural competence is an ethical responsibility (La Framboise & Foster, 1989). To be contextually relevant, South African therapists need to develop the ability to work within participatory-democratic frameworks, share responsibility, use expertise as a resource rather than as a distancing factor, tolerate ambiguity, demonstrate flexibility with clients, and take cognizance of broader social structures (Lazarus, 1985).

The Professional Board for Psychology in South Africa has recommended, but not insisted on, cross-cultural training for psychologists (Kriegler, 1993). Kriegler states that: "Much of the problem resides in the lack of direction and the tedious process of developing new programs, especially as universities are already under considerable stress and staff overloaded with research responsibilities (although much of the research does not escape the same criticism as pertains to training)" (p. 65).

A danger of transcultural psychology in South Africa is that it can operate from a series of disparaging assumptions concerning the apparently bizarre or the "otherness" of supposedly discrete groups (Swartz, 1987, p. 27). A veneer of cultural tolerance in cross-cultural psychology may express goodwill, "while the practise of tolerance means that other cultures are scrutinized, categorized, labeled, and assessed by dominant norms and values" (Essed, 1991, p. 211). Cross-cultural perspectives have been criticized for depicting stereotypes and caricatures of individuals (Hickson & Kriegler, 1996, p. 9), and some professionals have preferred to focus on the universality of suffering and confusion as a nondivisive strategy.

The implication that one culture is better than another has led Pedersen (1988) to advocate the use of the term "multicultural" counseling as opposed to "transcultural," "cross-cultural" or "intercultural" counseling. Pedersen (1991) has recognized the importance of counselor sensitivity to culture, but distinguished the multicultural revolution in counseling from exotic evaluations in which the culturally different are patronizingly treated as curiosities or as inferior: "We are moving toward a generic theory of multiculturalism as a "fourth force" position. Complimenting the other three forces of psychodynamic, behavioral and humanistic explanations of human behavior, the label of fourth force emphasizes that multiculturalism is relevant throughout the field of counseling as a generic rather than an exotic perspective" (1991, p. 6).

Given South Africa's history, there is a danger in emphasizing separatism in ways that are divisive and disunifying (Hickson & Kriegler, p. 5). The multicultural perspective "combines the extremes of relativism by explaining behavior both in terms of those culturally learnt perspectives that are unique to a particular culture and in the search for common ground universals that are shared across cultures" (Pedersen, 1991, p. 6). This perspective acknowledges that: "We are each like other people, like some other people, and like no other person" (Pedersen & Leong, 1997, p. 117).

The sameness–difference dilemma confronting South African psychology links to tensions between emic and etic perspectives. Pedersen (1998) poses the question whether the therapist should emphasize the culturally unique (emic) or the humanly universal (etic). If the cultural element is underemphasized, the counselor will be insensitive to the client's values; if it is overemphasized, the counselor will stereotype clients (Pedersen, 1998, p. 166). The challenge to practitioners venturing beyond their own cultural milieu "is how to strike a balance between the universal and the culturally specific, and how to switch from one frame of reference to the other, or how to combine the two" (Draguns, 1989, p. 21).

South African mental health practitioners are faced with the need to discern the location of their professions with reference to the rapidly changing nature of their country's social structures, and to rectify their past reliance on constructions that have not emerged from Africa (Drower, 2002). While organized psychology was encapsulated during the apartheid period there were other systems such as alternative therapies, tribal rituals, church and religious groups that might well have served a psychological function to fill in the vacuum left by encapsulated psychology. South Africa has commenced a process of reconstruction and development that both acknowledges its ancient African roots and heritage and incorporates the valuable contributions and traditions of its diverse population (Drower, 2002). Certain authors have posited the existence of an "African" psyche that require wholly different theoretical explications and thus different modes of psychological training if psychologists are to respond to broad mental health problems effectively. However, there are reservations concerning the role that unqualified multiculturalism should play in South African psychology. These reservations stem from perceptions of the microscopic examination of cultural difference in cross-cultural psychology in a manner similar to that that informed apartheid's vision. Freeman (1991) asserts that the call for an Afrocentric psychology glorified the so-called primitive, emphasizing an indigenous framework that reifies culture. Moreover, pejorative overtones of the commonly referred to First-Third world split often disempowers psychologists who readily come to believe that they have nothing of value to offer (Nell, 1990). There are, therefore, those such as Moll (2002) and Hountondji (1983) who argue that there is not a coherent psychological theory that is particular to Africa, but that a universal psychology engaged with the problems and issues of Africa and psychologists in Africa "can simultaneously extend the knowledge we have of humanity on our continent *and* help to transcend the narrow perspectives of dominant European and American psychological theory" (p. 13).

In South Africa, the notion of "cultural difference" provided an ideological basis and justification for political, mental, and socio-economic abuses during the apartheid era (L. Swartz, 1999). The patronizing apartheid policy of ascribing characteristics to certain groups without first consulting them, made many progressively-minded psychologists in South Africa wary of investigating real differences that may exist in a plural society. The assumption of these psychologists (e.g., Seedat, 1990; Seedat & Nell, 1990) has been that finding differences between groups served to justify their separateness, or the system of apartheid, and undermines the democratic initiative. However, little benefit seems to have been derived from working with knowledge that is censored or based on particular "criteria from within the realm of political rhetoric" (Swartz et al. cited in Kottler, 1990, p. 33). This approach moves researchers in the social sciences away from two important aims of critical theory and hermeneutic enquiry: first, a need to change society but also to be reflexive about its own status and that of its interpreter categories; and second, a critical examination of all fore-knowledge of the world and the phenomena we encounter there (Kottler, 1990, p. 33).

Many times well-meaning therapists have been guilty of cultural oppression because of their ignorance of the cultural norms of the diverse groups they were counseling. An understanding of the mismatch between Western psychotherapies and local cultural perspectives, and how multicultural practices may contradict, conflict, or coalesce with power determinants, can yield important information for the development of appropriate counseling techniques. In South Africa, the effects of racism and sexism, tribal traditions, deference relationships, and culture need not be seen in isolation. Trying to unravel their interactional effects may be difficult but beneficial (Hickson & Strous, 1993). A contribution of South African scholarship to the multicultural literature is its critical insistence on locating the construction of culture within an ideological context (Naidoo, 2000).

The affirmation of the value and distinctiveness of a group is frequently an aspect of liberatory struggles (Richards, 1997, p. xii). It is pragmatically important for oppressed people to reclaim and assert their difference in order for self-respect, dignity, and a real sense of identity to be acquired (Richards, 1997, p. 145). Tendencies to deny difference have often led to "color-blind racism" in which White cultural norms are proffered, and differences pathologized as deviant. A balance between a focus on differences and a focus on similarities both acknowledges specific cultural needs and affirms common humanity (Hickson & Kriegler, 1996; Richards, 1997, p. 306).

Resistance to cultural psychology reflects indignant reactions to the cross-cultural study of Blacks within a pejorative deficit model (Greene, 1985). The multicultural movement eschews the trend in social science to treat cultural differences as deficits. The multicultural acknowledgement of difference and emphasis on cultural sensitivity training acknowledges that no culture is superior to another.

Because human and cultural diversity are at the very core of psychology, a multicultural perspective might celebrate rather than be threatened by cultural diversity (Bodibe, 1993). The rehabilitation of multicultural psychology has been called for as a critical imperative for South African psychology (Nell, 1993).

The acceptance of human diversity is a value that promotes respect and appreciation (Prilleltensky, 1997). Granting individuals the opportunity to define their own identity produces salutary effects. Nonrecognition or misrecognition of identity can be a form of harmful oppression, which occurs when vulnerable groups are subjected to pejorative constructions by more powerful social agents (Prilleltensky, p. 522). Multicultural counseling may thus provide a nonracist, antisubjugatory basis for psychology (Nell, 1993).

SUMMARY

Cultural diversity, equality, and nondiscrimination are recursive themes in human rights literature. Human rights provisions that focus on inclusionary group participation and nondiscrimination offer a contraposition to exclusionary mental health practices that stereotype Blacks and stigmatize the mentally ill. The importation of a human rights culture to mental health could help to conscientize practitioners to the need for racial sensitivity and multicultural skills.

Nonelitism and collaborative consultation underpin attempts to democratize psychotherapy. Democracy presupposes a world in which one acts with people rather than on their behalf (Louw, 1983). Literature on the Working Alliance, phenomenological and existential psychotherapy, systemic therapy and critical family therapy, community psychology, and multicultural counseling are all replete with themes of diversity, respect, personal and group rights, empowerment, nonsubjugation, self-determination, and collaboration.

Recognition of the need to limit authoritarianism and elitism in psychology dovetail with the human rights approach to limitations on executive authorities. The notion of self-determination in psychology and in psychotherapy takes on board discourses of participatory democracy embraced in discussions on human rights.

Having covered literature relating to mental health and human rights, therapeutic relationships, community psychology, and multicultural counseling, the somewhat less directly related philosophical contribution of postmodernism will be addressed in the next chapter. As noted by Pedersen (1999), more recent characterizations of multiculturalism have been influenced by postmodernism's emphasis on understanding and description rather than causation, interpretation rather than statistical analysis, language, discourse, and symbols rather than reductionism, cultural contexts rather than context-free perspectives, and subjectivity rather than objectivity.

5

Postmodernism, Social Constructionism, and Their Confluence with Democratic Ideals

Postmodernism and social constructionism recognize that historical and evaluative contexts invalidate the notion of "value-free" research. Postmodern discussions rage about the nature of truth and who has authority to claim knowledge (L. Swartz, 1998). In contradistinction to what have been termed "hegemonic" voices and colonial voices having authority about what is and is not said about the world, postmodernism thrives on ideas about plurality of experience, multiple interpretations, and subaltern voices—such as voices of women, the formerly colonized, and sexual and racial minorities (Jordan & Weedon, 1995; L. Swartz, 1998, p. 238).

Postmodernism derives from disenchantment with the project of modernity, which sough to capture the nature of reality in self-enclosed theoretical systems or metanarratives, and to thus render knowledge universal and value-free (Painter & Theron, 1998). Recognition that power is integral to the production of knowledge has led to postmodern and social constructionist enquiries regarding the function of science as a tool of domination, legitimizing oppressive discourses (Prilleltensky, 1997, p. 527). In response to the limitations of positivism in the social sciences, postmodernism challenges the most fundamental foundations of modern science. Postmodernists have thus

questioned the notion of a knowable reality by emphasizing the socio-historical and political nature of all knowledge claims. By analyzing the socio-historical determinants of concepts and theories, especially those in the social sciences, postmodern analysts have been able to demonstrate how specialist disciplines of knowledge maintain and reproduce the dominant social relations and institutions of society; relations and institutions which are shaped by capitalism, patriarchy and racism. (Augoustinos & Walker, cited in Eagle, 1998)

Social-constructionist science studies critique the received view of science (Woolgar, 1996). The degree to which a given account of the world or self is sustained across time is viewed as not dependent on the objective validity of the account but on the vicissitudes of social process (Gergen, 1994, p. 126). Constructionists are deeply committed to the view that what we take to be objective knowledge and truth is the result of perspective. Constructionists contend that, "contrary to commonsense, there is no unique 'real world' that pre-exists and is independent of human mental activity and human symbolic language" (Bruner, cited by Schwandt, 1998, p. 125). Knowledge and truth are thus created rather than discovered by mind (Schwandt, 1998).

The postmodern ethic of pluralistic experience facilitates multicultural respect and tolerance through avoiding the reproduction of diversity into systems of ideological closure (Painter & Theron, 1998). Pedersen and Ivey (1993) link their culture-centered approach to counseling to the constructionist perspective, based on the premise that there is no directly accessible, singular, stable, and fully knowable external reality, but rather culturally embedded, interpersonally connected, and necessarily limited perspectives of reality (McNamee & Gergen, 1992). Reality, according to this view, is based not on an absolute truth but on complex and dynamic relationships in a cultural context (Pedersen, 1997).

FOUCAULDIAN PERSPECTIVES

According to Michel Foucault (1976), practices of modern power insidiously construct dominant "truths" that incite persons to embrace their own subjugation. For instance, Foucault holds that psychiatric institutions, and their attendant diagnostic systems, succeed in creating an autonomous sub-class of psychological deviants; and by concentrating the unusual behavior that threatens the mass of the population in one group, contain it. The existence of a confined and highly visible class of socially isolated patients, and the threat to members of the public that if they behave inappropriately they may join that class, allows for the social control of aberrant behavior. This analysis suggests the induction of individuals in the policing of their own behavior; a ruse that ensures our collusion in the specification of lives according to the dominant knowledges of our culture (White, 1991).

Following a Foucauldian line of argument, Littlewood and Lipsedge (1997) contend that both the Black and the mentally ill have been castigated as aliens in order to provide a model for the rest of society as to how *not* to be. According to this argument, labeling Blacks and the mentally ill as "deficient" serves to legitimize the existing order. Blacks and the mentally ill could constitute a challenge to prevailing norms based on dominant White values. Unfavorably contrasting their humanity with the supposed humanity of the predominant White norm, legitimizes the status quo. Blacks and the mentally ill provide a model of outsider, "not us" to the average individual. The outsider, as deficient alien, defines the limits of normality by producing boundaries only within which normality is achievable (Littlewood & Lipsedge, 1997).

The coherence of racism and victimization of the mentally ill was, arguably, most apparent in Nazi ideology. Mentally ill and retarded Germans were an embarrassment to the Nazi concept of a super race. The "euthanasia" of mentally ill persons and the systematic murder of homosexuals, political opponents, Gypsies, and millions of Jews stemmed from grossly misanthropic intolerance concerning "nonAryans."

In identifying the major function of the "outsider" as being to promote individual adaptation, Littlewood and Lipsedge (1997, p. 29) refer to the psychoanalytic notion of projection. Psychoanalysis suggests that we scapegoat others by projecting onto them our own unacceptable impulses. The outsider is often portrayed as dirty, bestial, aggressive, treacherous, stupid, and sexually voracious.

The argument that others are fundamentally different provides a rationale for keeping them separated or alienated from mainstream society. Apartheid in South Africa, ghettoisation around the world, and the establishment of mental institutions attest to the often isolated and alienated position of both Blacks and the mentally ill in society. Psychologists habitually espouse a commitment to client empowerment. Yet, the mental health profession has been slated for perpetuating negative stereotypes of Blacks as well as for stigmatizing the mentally ill. A Black person in need of mental health services may be in double jeopardy because of potential shortcomings in the mental health system and the potential perpetuation of racial discrimination within that system.

An historical analysis of psychology might reveal not only the benefits it has to offer in the promotion of mental health, but also how it binds us (Louw, 2002). For example, psychology can be used to manage people in large numbers. When people are gathered in large numbers in one "plane of sight," individual differences become more visible (Rose, 1988). Individuals might then be expected to regulate themselves in accordance with what Foucault described as "technologies of the self," to moderate themselves "in relation to the true and the false, the permitted and the forbidden, the desirable and the undesirable" (1988, p 144).

By failing to take cognizance of the content of those behavioral norms that it so readily accepts, the mental health profession tends to tacitly accept the status quo and to ignore those stresses existing in what may be a pathological social environment. Within the context of medical power, oppressed people have perceived health care systems as an extension of their disempowerment by the state (Seedat & Nell, 1992). Foucault's writings (1965, 1976, 1990) raise the issue of professional psychology and psychiatry's complicity in undemocratic practices. The goal of democratic society is to maximize the quality of life for all, while limiting the extent to which its constituents are subjected to social control methods (Arrigo & Williams, 1999). From a Foucauldian perspective, mental health treatment runs the risk of fostering subjugation by sacrificing diversity "at the altar of medical knowledge" (Arrigo & Williams, p. 178).

DECONSTRUCTION

The social constructionist position offers the possibility of research for emancipatory purposes (Prilleltensky, 1997). Deconstructive methods may be used to uncover oppressive messages inherent in social, cultural, and scientific discourses, and in the hands of oppressed individuals can help to challenge illegitimate structures of authority (Burman & Parker, 1993). Adherents of an affirmative school of postmodernism embrace a political agenda similar to empowerment (Prilleltensky, 1997, p. 528; Rosenau, 1992), whereas adherents of a skeptical trend in postmodernism (Rosenau, 1992) are wary of political activism because of their reluctance to make normative pronouncements that are potentially dogmatic. The creation of frameworks sensitive to context and to people's voices may counter the objection of skeptical postmodernism to moral postulates that pretend to speak to and for all people (Prilleltensky, 1997, p. 528).

Deconstruction, according to Michael White's definition:

has to do with procedures that subvert taken-for-granted realities and practices; these so-called "truths" that are split off from the conditions and the context of their production, those disembodied ways of speaking that hide their biases and prejudices, and those familiar practices of self and of relationship that are subjugating of person's lives. Many of the methods of deconstruction render strange these familiar and everyday taken-for-granted realities and practices by objectifying them. In this sense, the methods of deconstruction are methods that "exoticize the domestic." (1991, p. 121)

Deconstruction is an intensely critical mode of unraveling how systems of meaning lure people into taking certain notions for granted and privileging certain ways of being over others (Parker, 1999). The deconstructive task is to locate a problem in certain cultural practices and to comprehend the role of patterns of power in setting out positions for people that serve to reinforce the idea that they can do nothing about it themselves (Parker, p. 3).

DISCOURSE ANALYSIS

Emphasis on the deconstruction of social discourse has given rise to attempts to gain understanding of social life and social interaction from a study of social texts (Potter & Wetherell, 1992). Foucault (1972) and Parker (1992) following Foucault have conceptualized discourses as statements or practices that construct the objects of which they speak (Coyle, 1995).

Discourse analysis is a qualitative research methodology that subjects spoken and written material to textual analysis in order to uncover how language not only reflects but also constructs social life. It examines how people use language to construct versions of their worlds and what they gain from these constructions:

Discourse analysis can reveal the constructed nature and the implications of oppressive discourses and can emphasize that alternative nonoppressive discourses can be constructed in their place. Discourse analysis assumes that all linguistic material has **action orientation**, that is, it is used to perform particular social functions such as justifying, questioning and accusing, and it achieves this by employing a variety of rhetorical strategies. Key tasks that discourse analysts set themselves are to identify what functions are being performed by the linguistic material that is being analyzed and to consider how these functions are performed. This entails a close and careful inspection of the text. (Coyle, 1995, p. 245)

The following semi-tongue-in-cheek appraisal of how talk is deconstructed to reveal action orientation is provided by Charles Antaki (2000): "Once you start looking closely at what people do, you can never go back to cramming them into categories or treating their words as printouts. It does mean hours spent hunched over the tape-recorder or the video screen, but the dividends are enormous. And if the psychologist is a nosy parker interested in what people do with each other, there can't be more profitable fun than that" (p. 243).

For Parker (1992), discourses function to legitimate and buttress existing institutions, reproduce power relations and inequities in society, and have ideological effects. The study of racism has proven fertile ground for the study of discourse, or what Potter & Wetherell (1992) call "interpretive repertoires." Discourse analysis has become increasingly popular in the study of racism as ideology (Miles, 1989; Stevens, 1998; van Dijk, 1991). Discourse analysis is also one of the research methodologies used to critically reflect on the political import of social psychological theory and research (Painter & Theron, 1998).

REFLEXIVITY AND CRITICAL THEORY

Reflexivity was described by Mead (1934) as "the turning back of the experience of the individual upon [her-himself]" (p. 134) and by Delamont (1991) as "a social-scientific variety of self-consciousness" (cited in King, 1996, pp. 175-176). Reflexivity is based on an understanding that researchers' accounts of how the language used by people is constructed are themselves constructions (Potter & Wetherell, 1992). Professional disciplines have developed language practices and techniques that encourage belief that members of these disciplines have access to objective and unbiased accounts of reality (White, 1991): "What this means is that certain speakers, those with training in certain special techniques—supposedly to do with the powers of the mind to make contact with reality—are privileged to speak with authority beyond the range of their personal experience" (Parker & Shotter, cited by White, 1991, p. 142).

Built-in injunctions against querying the contextual validity of expert opinion make it difficult if not impossible for others to engage in dialogue over different points of view (White, 1991, p. 143). Self-reflexively uncovering the socially constructed nature of social psychological explanations and showing how these explanations reproduce and maintain social power relations rather than represent neutral reality has been a key focus of critical social psychology (Henriques, Holway, Urwin, & Walkerdine, 1984; Ibanez & Iniquez, 1997; Painter & Theron, 1998; Wexler, 1983). The goal of critical theory is emancipatory discourse, "attained by initiating a process of self-reflection in those subjects whose self-formative capacity is radically truncated by the constraints of ideological forms of consciousness" (Ivey, 1986, p. 7).

Ideology, as a pattern of both factual and normative beliefs and concepts that purport to explain complex social phenomena, directs and simplifies social political choices (Carlton, 1977; Dawes, 1985). For Heather (1976), ideological self-interest:

is not something of which its exponents are necessarily aware, and ideology does not refer to an overt "conspiracy" on the part of capitalists to prolong their exploitation. Rather, their exploitation is protected by a system of illusions which serve to make it appear legitimate and disguise its true nature. The exploiters are just as much victims of these illusions as those they exploit, since their self-interest also prevents them from realizing the character of their exploitative relationships with others. (pp. 42–43)

While psychology has been seen to operate independently of the political realm as a "value-free science," those who would contextualize the discipline (e.g., Ingleby, 1981) see the goal of uncontaminated truth as mystifying, owing to our inability to escape the history of everyday social categories. Social scientists such as psychologists are exposed to politicking just as are other citizens, and can be rendered unconscious of false elements in what they come to accept as natural (Dawes, 1985): "When we operate with lack of awareness of the ideological influences in our work, we can believe passionately that we are dealing with truth. This lack of awareness can lead us to play a role (unwittingly) in exploiting our discoveries of what is natural about a social or psychological phenomenon, to support a particular social order" (Ingleby, 1974, cited by Dawes, 1985).

The goal of critical theory as an emancipatory science is the initiation of self-reflection in ideologically constrained persons (Ivey, 1986): "Critically informed self-reflection results in subjects attaining insight into their once ideologically obscured circumstances of domination. Such insight serves to dissolve the quasi-causal hold of ideology on human agency, thus freeing individuals *from* rigidified patterns of thought and action and freeing *for* new rationally considered socio-political praxis. Ideology critique thus ideally results in a restoration of the interrupted individual and collective self-formative process" (pp. 8–9).

Research in the critical tradition takes the form of self-conscious criticism where researchers try to become aware of the ideological imperatives that inform their research. Thus, critical researchers enter into an investigation with their assumptions on the table (Kincheloe & McLaren, 1998): "Whereas traditional researchers cling to the guard-rail of neutrality, critical researchers frequently announce their partisanship in the struggle for a better world" (Kincheloe & McLaren, p. 140).

Calls for reflexivity within postmodernism and social constructionism have had their major impact in the areas of qualitative research. A number of psychotherapies also reflect postmodernist and poststructuralist underpinnings. Critical movements in the deconstruction of power in therapy are concerned to understand how we come to occupy certain standpoints. "This is where a concern for justice in therapy becomes intertwined with a concern for social justice in the world" (Parker, 1999, p. 4). Michael White's systemic narrative approach, for instance, helps clients to self-reflexively find unique outcomes to contradict self-subjugatory dominant narratives. Psychodynamic notions of transference and countertransference have also been affected by calls for reflexivity in social science research and practice.

TRANSFERENCE-COUNTERTRANSFERENCE PHENOMENA

One of the strongest recognitions that therapists are neither dispassionate observers of human behavior, nor capable of objective analyses untainted by personal constructs, is to be found in transference and countertransference literature (e.g., Brabender, 1987; Pollack & Levy, 1989; Racker, 1957). A social constructionist approach has influenced psychodynamic notions of transference–countertransference phenomena, which are seen as key issues in the understanding of counselor–client interactions. The development of relational understandings of transference and countertransference (Greenberg & Mitchell, 1983) resonate with postmodern calls for reflexivity. The issues of transference and countertransference will be discussed here because they draw attention to the fact that psychological endeavors do not occur in objectively controlled environments. Psychotherapy and interracial therapy occur within the context of client and therapist constructions of reality and meaning.

Transference

There is a large body of literature on the subject of transference. For our purposes, transference may be considered a form of projection from client to therapist (Carter, 1995, p. 18). A definition used by many clinicians states that: "Transference is the experiencing of feelings, drives, attitudes, fantasies and defenses towards a person in the present which are inappropriate to that person and are a repetition, a displacement of reactions originating in regard to significant persons of early childhood" (Greenson, 1965, cited by Carter, p. 18).

Sigmund Freud identified transference as occurring whenever patients displace to a therapist feelings of love or hate that they had previously attached to a significant person. The concept of transference has since been broadened by a number of psychoanalysts, including Melanie Klein. Klein (1948) suggested that people project transference relationships into virtually every activity. Her conceptualization has resulted in the recognition of transference as operating in a multiplicity of situations. The word "transference" has come to be used rather loosely by many therapists for any feelings that the patient may have for the therapist (Malan, 1979, p. 68). Transference also plays out in overt interpersonal behavior in conversations between strangers (Andersen & Miranda, 2000). All these understandings of transference have clear implications for working in multicultural and interracial relationships.

Deficit models of Black personality or cultural misunderstandings may predispose White therapists to misinterpret transference phenomena in interracial contexts. Therapy-undermining reactions by clients may be attributed by therapists to poor or aberrant ego functioning, uncontrollable id impulses or an unrestrained superego, rather than to racially based discrimination and social oppression previously experienced by Black patients (Carter, 1995, p. 36). Therapists should be open to the possibility that a client's defensiveness may result not from neurosis but from rational negative reactions to the therapist's bigotry or stereotyping: "Disturbed, unhealthy responses of the patient in the therapeutic situation cannot ... be assumed to be necessarily transference phenomena. They may be 'pseudo-transference' responses to unhealthy attitudes or behavior of the therapist, and therefore not an accurate reflection of the patient's neurosis. The well-known countertransference phenomena caused by an unhealthy pattern of individual origin in the therapist can produce such pseudo-transference reactions" (Thomas, 1962, p. 899).

Countertransference

As with the concept of transference, the theoretical understanding of "countertransference" has grown and expanded. According to Carter: "Countertransference is the flipside of transference, wherein the therapist's own unconscious feelings, thoughts, and actions are stimulated by the therapeutic material .... Most would agree that countertransference refers to the manner in which the therapist's own life experience and personality influences the therapeutic process" (1995, p. 17).

Initially, Sigmund Freud regarded countertransference as an obstruction to the psychoanalyst's understanding of the patient. He thought of the analyst's mind as an interpretation instrument, which loses its accuracy when countertransference interferes (Sandler, Holder, & Dare, 1970). His view of countertransference was as a sort of resistance in the analyst toward a patient, due to the arousal of unconscious conflicts elicited by the patient. Countertransference might arise when an analyst was unable to deal appropriately with aspects of the patient's communication and behavior because they impinged on the analyst's own inner problems. Freud was of the opinion that analysts should themselves undergo periodic analysis in order to gain insight and to overcome psychological deficiencies caused by such unresolved unconscious conflicts.

Freud's formulation of countertransference as an obstacle to the analytic work has resulted in many psychotherapists taking the view that countertransference is unwelcome in therapy sessions. Weigert (1954, p. 243) spoke of a "countertransference tabu," exemplified in the attitude that "the analyst must not have countertransference reactions" (Moosa, 1992). A countertransference-as-hindrance model, which views countertransference as an impediment, rises out of the modernist drive/structure model of psychoanalysis, wherein detachment is seen as a prerequisite for objectivity (Peebles-Kleiger, 1989). In early psychoanalytic conceptualizations, the therapist was meant to remain objective and to serve as a screen onto which the patient was free to project and thus reveal the drama and dramatis personae from the past. By observing what was being projected, the therapist could discover what the patient must have experienced (Peebles-Kleiger, 1989, p. 520). This drive/structure model based on nineteenth century Cartesian scientific philosophy, conceptualized the therapist as standing outside the emotional field of patients to achieve the greatest clarity of vision (Greenberg & Mitchell, 1983). Countertransference was seen to arise solely from the therapist's unresolved conflicts, and was seen to have the power to distort the therapist's reading of the projected picture and to contaminate the picture itself (Peebles-Kleiger, 1989).

In contradiction to the countertransference-as-hindrance model, a countertransference-as-facilitator model recognizes the utility of countertransference in sessions (Peebles-Kleiger, 1989). Countertransference, in the latter model, is recognized as supplying important information for the therapist. A major development in psychoanalytic writings on countertransference has been the idea that the analyst has unconscious access to elements of understanding and appreciation of processes occurring in the patient, which are not immediately consciously available to the analyst. These elements can be discovered if the analyst monitors his or her own mental associations while listening to the patient (Heinmann, 1950, 1960; Sandler et al., 1970).

In the countertransference-as-facilitator model, feelings toward the patient are regarded as inevitable aspects of the interaction, rather than as by-products of unresolved therapist conflicts. The therapist learns about the patient as an involved participant, attentive to his or her own countertransference issues, rather than as a dispassionate observer who has successfully overcome countertransference issues. Countertransference is no longer regarded as the warp in the screen; in some ways, it is the screen itself (Peebles-Kleiger, p. 520).

The countertransference-as-facilitator model is compatible with what Greenberg and Mitchell (1983) identify as the relational/structure model in psychoanalytic thought. The poststructuralist relational model recognizes that therapists and clients influence one another. It is based on twentieth century field theories (e.g., Heisenberg & Einstein), which recognize that there is no absolute truth available to scientist observers. The scientist-practitioner is unavoidably involved with the observed in the relational field. This view is in keeping with the postmodern concept of "relativity of knowledge;" that truth is mediated by the person observing it.

Peebles-Kleiger (1989) point out three reasons why therapists have been reluctant to adopt the relational/structure model despite the potential usefulness of being mindful of one's own countertransference reactions:

1.   The drive and relational models represent alternative paradigms. A move to the relational model can create untenable dissonance and loyalty conflicts in therapists who

have been trained, treated, and supervised in a traditional psychoanalytic drive/structure model. (Greenberg & Mitchell (1983) contend that "model mixing," the juxtaposing of drive and relational models, leads to unstable metamodels because each of these models makes absolute claims based on incommensurable *a priori* premises. According to this line of argument, a therapist must ultimately choose implicitly or explicitly between the relational or drive paradigms.)

2. The goal of protecting the client has promoted the study of countertransference to uncover the analyst's pathology (Epstein & Feiner, 1979) and has helped inhibit adoption of the relational/structure model of countertransference.

3. Anxiety accompanies our discovery of primitive impulses and processes in ourselves, and, as a result, we repress feared impulses. A circumscribed focus on the patient's emotions alone is sometimes an effort to preserve the therapist's own emotional resources (pp. 521–522).

Despite objections to the relational model's view of countertransference, the countertransference-as-facilitator model, which is compatible with postmodern understandings, has proven popular. The countertransference taboo may encourage a phobic attitude in the analyst towards his or her own emotional reactions, thus limiting understanding of the patient (Kernberg, 1974). Several writers have broadened the concept of countertransference to include the totality of the therapist's conscious and unconscious relations to both the patient's and the therapist's transferential and reality needs (Little, 1951; Searles, 1965; Weigert, 1954; Winnicott, 1949 and more recently, Boyer, 1989; Brabender, 1987; Carpy, 1989; Pollack & Levy, 1989). Postmodernist and social constructionist appeals for reflexivity have encouraged researchers and therapists to become aware of their feelings, biases, and personal peccadilloes and to scrutinize these closely (King, 1996).

A definition of countertransference as the therapist's total range of feelings for and against the patient was largely facilitated by Melanie Klein's (1946) description of the process of projective identification (Moosa, 1992). Racker (1957) subsequently introduced the term "complimentary countertransference," which has in common with projective identification the process where the therapist unwittingly identifies with or experiences the feelings of significant people in the patient's past who have been internalized by the patient and projected onto the therapist. Racker also introduced the term "concordant countertransference" to refer to therapist identification with the patient's self-representation. Implicit in these perspectives is the point that countertransference "does not always involve unresolved pathology; in many instances the analyst has his own realistic responses to his patient's realistically socially unacceptable, seductive or other behavior" (Kaplan & Sadock cited by Moosa, 1992, p. 128).

Concordant countertransference feelings have functional diagnostic value because they enable an understanding of patients' inarticulate experiences. The concept of empathic, or concordant identification (Racker, 1957) describes the process whereby the therapist identifies with the patient's feelings, which are invariably unconscious or conscious but difficult for the patient to verbalize. This process is analogous to feelings of empathy, in which the therapist is closely attuned to emotions the patient is experiencing. The therapist's complimentary countertransference reactions also have diagnostic value in allowing him or her to understand how people close to the patient have responded to the patient. Nonrecognition of complimentary countertransference could lead to potential errors in therapy (Moosa, 1992).

Moosa (1992), in a paper concerned with countertransference in overtly political trauma work in South Africa, calls upon South African therapists to be more conscious of the role of countertransference, for better or worse, in their work with traumatized individuals. Some of the countertransference themes that emerged from her study, linked to feelings of demoralization, anger, guilt, value conflicts, and self-protection, are likely to present themselves in interracial counseling contexts to varying degrees.

Moosa's study (1992) dealt with the intense countertransference reactions of therapists working with victims of political repression. The countertransference reactions of therapists in less violent contexts may be less intense and not as easily detected. Countertransference issues of demoralization, anger, value conflict, self-protection, and guilt are nevertheless likely to manifest in interracial counseling contexts to some degree even when clients have not been victimized as immediately or intensely as in Moosa's study. A lengthy history of racism and oppression has dominated the political terrain of South Africa and left its mark on the mental health system, counselors, and clients. Negative counselor reactions to Blacks, or even placatory attitudes on the part of counselors, may threaten the Working Alliance as well as dialogical or phenomenological exploration (Cooper, 1973; Greene, 1995; Heine, 1950; Jackson, 1973; Jones & Seagull, 1977; Pinderhughes, 1973; Ridley, 1995; Vontress, 1971). The therapy-hindering effects of counselor countertransference, as well as its beneficial therapy-facilitating effects need to be understood. Constant scrutiny by the analyst of variations in his or her countertransference feelings and attitudes towards the patient can lead to increased insight into processes occurring in the patient (Sandler et al., 1970, p. 87).

The pertinence of countertransference reactions in interracial therapy is that White counselors frequently perceive Black clients in the same manner as they perceive Blacks in general (Vontress, 1971): "It is important for the white counselor to acknowledge racial feelings and attitudes he brings to any counseling interview he conducts with blacks. As a product of a racist society, he perforce brings to that relationship certain ideas and attitudes" (p. 9).

Counselors are frequently unaware of their own racial attitudes. Ridley (1995) offers the following reasons as to why White therapists pervasively act in a manner that suggests imperviousness to racial issues:

1. Counselors may have a strong need to appear impartial, fearing that they are unconscious bigots deep down.
2. Counselors may feel race is a sensitive and uncomfortable topic to discuss, or they may have insecurities or unresolved personal issues about race.
3. Some counselors are overprotective of their clients and try not to hurt them.
4. Some counselors hide their lack of knowledge of racial issues by not discussing them (pp. 67–68).

Apart from the diagnostic value of countertransference attunement, some writers have focused on therapeutic benefits to be derived from proper management of the countertransference. How the therapist reacts to what is stirred within serves as a model for the patient struggling to handle similar feelings (Peebles-Kleiger, 1989). Pines (1986) described how one patient "needed to test my capacity to express her affects for her until she was strong enough to feel them herself" (cited by Peebles-Kleiger, 1989, p. 522). This use of countertransference is akin to Bion's (1957) concept of the therapist as a container and metabolizer of affects the patient cannot yet metabolize and thus integrate into the self. Herzog (1984, cited by Peebles-Kleiger, p. 523) has noted that patients ultimately learn to become effective interrogators of their own experience by watching their therapists synthesize and integrate not only the various affects experienced by their patients, but also the affects stirred in themselves. In similar vein, Hamilton (1992) has proposed that: "What is conveyed to the patient is both the transformed, original projection from the patient and an aspect of the analyst's self—the containing aspect of the analyst, the analyzing function itself—which he wishes, however benignly and gently, to insinuate into the patient so as to influence him" (pp. 166–167).

While countertransference can be employed positively, the unconscious acting out of countertransference inevitably has a destructive impact on therapy (G. Ivey, 1992). Countertransference pathology is testimony to the fact that therapists, in spite of their training, are simply human beings, subject to the same needs, desires, and failings as anyone else. The situation is compounded by cognitive and humanistic orientations that inadvertently foster countertransference pathology and do not provide a framework for its detection and rectification (G. Ivey, 1992).

Therapists' awareness of their own and of their clients' intrapsychic and interpersonal dynamics are critical if deleterious countertransference reactions are to be managed and if beneficial countertransference reactions are to be positively harnessed." The notion that a psychoanalyst would have an active, if sometimes unconscious, intention to influence or insinuate an aspect of his or her own self-experience into the patient, even while adopting a neutral and interpretative stance, goes further in the direction of acknowledging that the therapist is always an active presence, even when he or she is quiet" (Hamilton, 1992, p. 163).

Postmodern and social constructionist viewpoints that there is no one observable truth but a multiplicity of constructed perspectives, and that researchers and the researched, as well as counselors and clients, influence each other's constructions further lend emphasis to the need to understand and appreciate the significance of both transference and countertransference phenomena. Such an endeavor may empower therapists to help their clients in enlightened and nonsubjugating ways.

SUMMARY

Social constructionist and postmodern perspectives facilitate counselor sensitivity to issues of race and racism by challenging taken-for-granted ideological positions and by challenging positivist assumptions. Researchers are encouraged to consult collaboratively with members of the groups they are researching rather than to assume automatic validity of research conclusions and superior knowledge on the part of the researcher. For example, discourse analysis shifts the prominence of researchers as experts in human beings and their behavior, to "experts...in the range of questions we can formulate, and interpretations we can access" (Billington, 1995, p 38).

Democratic principles are implicit in both social constructionist research and psychotherapies embracing a postmodern ethos. These approaches recognize that collaboration:

is necessary for the realization of self-determination, for individuals to assert their identities, and ultimately to feel part of the world around them. Inasmuch as this value enhances the level of connectedness among people, it contributes to a sense of community (Fox, 1993a, Frazer & Lacey, 1993). The dual purpose of collaboration and democratic participation is to express one's opinions and to create bonds of care while upholding personal rights and social responsibilities (Avineri & De Shalit, 1992; Bernstein, 1983; Etzioni, 1991, 1993; Habermas, 1990a, 1990b). (Prilleltensky, 1997, p. 527)

Critical theory recognizes the need for a more egalitarian and democratic reconstruction of the social sciences in particular and of society in general. In pursuit of these goals, deconstructive methods and emancipatory discourse are employed to try to liberate both professionals and members of disempowered groups from ideologically informed processes of domination. In psychotherapy, emphasis on critical reflexivity requires therapists to be aware of transference and countertransference phenomena, which amongst other impacts may either facilitate or hinder interracial counseling. The section that follows presents two models designed to sensitize counselors to the need to critically evaluate their own assumptions.

Part III

Training Models

This section describes the Triad Model for cultural sensitivity training and proposes a supplementary model for further research. Chapter 6 discusses the underlying assumptions of the Triad Model, the nature of Triad training, research on the Model, and its variants. Chapter 7 presents an Anticlient-Proclient Model. I use the term "anticlient" to refer to the often unspoken mindsets of counselors that are undermining of interracial and multicultural therapy, and the term "proclient" to refer to attitudes that are supportive of interracial and multicultural therapy. Drawing off the disparate anti and pro therapy influences mentioned in the first two sections of this book, I suggest that the Anticlient-Proclient Model holds promise for improved counselor sensitivity in interracial and multicultural counseling contexts. Although developed with reference to White South African counselors, the model could have generic relevance for all counselors, especially in contexts where counselors work with people from diverse cultural, social, or economic backgrounds. Chapter 8 reports on a study that gleaned benchmark descriptions of the anticlient position, the proclient position, their differences, the manner in which competing anticlient and proclient sentiments are negotiated, and implications for training with the Anticlient-Proclient Model.

6

Hearing Clients' Inner Talk in Multicultural Contexts: Pedersen's Triad Model

The Triad Model was developed by Paul Pedersen in order to train students in individual counseling with culturally diverse clients. The Triad Model has a multicultural focus, which acknowledges that, at least in the United States, the vast majority of clients receiving mental health services are nonWhite, from lower socio-economic levels, and differ significantly from counselors in their socialization and value assumptions.

According to Pedersen (1977; 1983; 1985; 1988; 1997; 2000), cultural background influences the way counseling is given and how it is received, but few opportunities exist for counselors to be trained for work with culturally different clients. Although clients make culturally informed value assumptions, there has been a lack of coordinated training in cultural sensitivity for mental health professionals. There is a tendency to assume that clients and counselors share the same value assumptions in spite of abundant evidence to the contrary. An assumption exists that counselors know the meaning of what is healthy and normal, when, in fact, they may merely be reflecting their own cultural encapsulation and political, social, or economic values. The constructs of healthy and normal which guide mental health services delivery are not the same across all cultures and might lend to culturally encapsulated counselors becoming a tool of particular political, social, or economic orders.

The multicultural focus that underpins the Triad Model has as its goal the increased understanding by counselors of diverse client groups and improved multicultural interventions. In Triad Model training, simulated counseling interviews and role-playing allow counselor trainees to make mistakes and learn recovery skills in multicultural contexts without risk to actual clients.

In its most basic form, this training model comprises a role-play between a counselor, a client, and an anticounselor. The anticounselor is a person selected from the client's cultural group and coached to role-play, in a simulated cross-cultural counseling interview, a personification of a client's problem. The anticounselor is deliberately subversive in attempting to disrupt the counseling interview and pulls in opposite direction to the counselor who is attempting to solve the problem. Through the supply of continuous and direct feedback to trainee counselors from the anticounselor, who personifies the change-resisting problem, sources of resistance in cross-cultural counseling are explicated. The trainee counselor thus receives immediate feedback as to his or her interventions that impede rapport in multicultural contexts, his or her inappropriate attempts to overcome client resistance, and how to deal with this.

While the anticounselor articulates the negative messages a client from a culture different to the trainee counselor's culture might be thinking but not saying, in more comprehensive training programs a procounselor role-player may be employed to explicate positive messages in a client's mind. An anticounselor or procounselor role-play may be used without its complement in training programs; while their combined use in extended programs helps trainee counselors hear the client's internal dialogue in both its positive and negative aspects. The assumption is that some client internal dialogue is positive and procounselor, while other inner messages are negative and anticounselor in orientation.

ASSUMPTIONS UNDERPINNING THE TRIAD MODEL

The Problem

The Triad Model describes counseling as a three-way interaction between a counselor, a client, and a problem from the client's perceptual worldview. Pedersen conceptualizes a problem as having the following characteristics:

1. Judging from the client's perspective, a problem has rewarding as well as punishing features. If the problem were unambiguously bad, the client would have an easier time disengaging.
2. A problem is complex, dynamic, ever changing and can elude simplistic labels.
3. A problem is active rather than passive, with an ability to change and constantly adapt.
4. A problem is not an abstraction, but from the client's point of view, is very concrete. It is defined by its own threats and promises in the perceptual worldview of the client.

That each problem has rewarding as well as punishing features presents a dilemma for the client. The problem is complex, like a personality, and not limited to a single presenting symptom. It changes actively, drawing its identity from the client's total environment of relationships. In counseling, the problem sometimes resembles a personified enemy with a secret strategy of its own.

A key element in the Triad Model is conceptualizing the balance of power between the counselor and client on the one hand, and the problem on the other. The unique element of Triad training is the personification of the problem in the anticounselor, who actively tries to prevent the counselor from coalescing with the client towards solving the problem. The problem is personified as if it were a third member of the counseling relationship.

The problem is perceived as belonging within the client's private world of phenomenological reality. If the counselor is to participate with the client in a coalition against the problem, he or she needs to accept the client's view of the problem as real even if only within the client's perceptual field. Accepting the client means accepting the problem as real and not ignoring the client's perception of reality. The client is seen as behaving as if the problem were true, and the problem is viewed as affecting both the client's and the counselor's behavior. The ultimate solution or desirable outcome assumes that the counselor and client are able to control the problem, to cope with its inhibiting effects, and to lessen its influence on the client's behavior.

The problem can be separated from the client in such a way that both the client and counselor can attack the problem without attacking the client. The client is not disassociated from the problem but recognizes the problem as a nonessential and inhibiting element of interaction with the environment. The problem is part of the client's perceptual field but is not an essential part of the client. The client's ability to define and distinguish the problem decreases its inhibiting effect, dissolves the problem-client coalition, and ensures that the client is no longer dominated by the problem (Pedersen, 2000b).

Counseling as a Coalition

According to Pedersen, counseling occurs in the context of equilibrium between the counselor seeking coalition with the client and the resistant nature of the problem. A pull-push forcefield exists in which the counselor seeks to be helpful, the client seeks to reconcile internalized ambiguity, and the problem seeks to continue controlling the client. The task function of counseling is to negotiate a coalition between the client and the counselor to balance the power influence of the problem. The greater the cultural disparity between the counselor and client, the less likely such a coalition will be established.

The effective counselor varies the power of intervention according to the client's changing needs. If a counselor assumes too much power, the client will withdraw from counseling in preference for the problem, which appears less threatening. If the counselor assumes too little power, the client will also withdraw to the problem from an ineffective counselor. Counselors might exert more power through confrontation and interpretation and less power through reflection and nondirective accommodation. To the extent that a counselor and client come from different cultures, it is particularly difficult to maintain the appropriate balance of power inside a counseling interview. The Triad Model provides a conceptual framework for operationalizing the counseling interaction and for defining the goal of training as increasing a counselor's skill in maintaining an effective, balanced relationship. The anticounselor tries to establish an alliance with the client against the counselor, while the procounselor tries to establish a client-counselor coalition against the problem. The anticounselor, representing the resistant nature of a problem, attempts to disrupt client-counselor problem solving endeavors.

Figure 1 outlines a schematic for describing the relationships between the counselor, client, and problem as a triadic interaction. This figure describes counseling as competition for power or influence between a client-counselor coalition on the one hand and the problem on the other. The client is expected to move up the slope from having less power to having more power as the desired outcome. The problem is expected to move down the slope from having more power to having less power as the desired outcome.

Figure 1
**A Schematic Description of the Ratio of Power Influence over Time for Counselor,
Counsellee and Problem with Three (X1, X2, X3) Points in the Counseling Process
Indicated (Pedersen, 2000b, p. 34)**

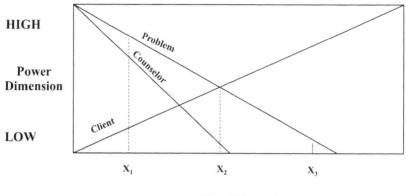

Time Dimension

At any given point along the time dimension, the power of the counselor plus the
power of the client should be equal to or greater than the power of the problem. The
counselor alone is always less powerful than the problem and this unequal distribution of power requires the counselor to vary the intensity of intervention accordingly.
Counselor interventions towards the left side of the schematic tend to be confronting
and interpretative while interventions toward the right side of the schematic tend to
be reflective and nondirective.

Three situations (X_1, X_2, X_3) are indicated on Figure 1. In X_1, the client has little
power and is dominated by the problem. Situation X_2 shows the client able to exert
enough power so that the counselor may become the weaker member of the triad,
transferring more responsibility to the client. Situation X_3 shows the client able to
manage the problem independently without help from the counselor.

The Notion of Self-Talk

The notion of client self-talk is fundamental to the Triad Model. Internal dialogue
(Meichenbaum, 1977) or self-talk (Ellis, 1962) may be characterized as talking to
one's self, usually in a two-sided or positive versus negative polarity. Credit for the
emergence of modern theoretical discussions of inner speech may be attributed to
Mead (1982) and symbolic interactional theory, as well as to sociocultural theory
articulated by Vygotsky (1962) and by Luria (1961).

In psychology, the term "inner speech" usually signifies soundless, mental speech, arising at
the instant we think about something, plan or solve problems in our mind, recall books read or
conversations heard, read and write silently. In all such instances we think and remember with
the aid of words that we articulate to ourselves. Inner speech is nothing but speech to oneself,
or concealed verbalization, which is instrumental to the logical processing of sensory data, in
their realization and comprehension within a definite system of concepts and judgments. The
elements of inner speech are found in all our conscious perceptions, actions and emotional

experiences, where they manifest themselves as verbal sets, instructions to oneself, or as verbal interpretation of sensations and perceptions. (Sokolov, 1972, p. 1)

Albert Ellis uses the term self-talk for internal dialogue in which people repeatedly utter internalized statements to themselves, while Beck (1976) describes internal dialogue as containing "automatic thoughts" because it seems to emerge automatically and rapidly. The self-statements, images, self-evaluations, and attributions that a person says, or fails to say, to him- or herself influences human behavior (Lange and Jacubowksi, 1976; Mahoney, 1974; Meichenbaum, 1974, 1975). According to Meichenbaum, the production of inner speech can "deautomize" behavior and provide the basis for new behavior. In his work with schizophrenics and with impulsive children, Meichenbaum (1974, 1975) has demonstrated an important relationship between a person's behavior and what that person says to him- or herself. Meichenbaum (1977) uses the term internal "dialogue" rather than internal "monologue" to suggest that one does not only speak to oneself, one also listens to oneself.

Inner or private speech is often associated with a dialogue between two sides, identities, or interactors, with one in a negative role and the other in a positive role. Even optimal thinking includes both positive and negative ideas, which provide a dialogical basis for thinking (Pedersen, 2000b; Swartz & Garamoni, 1989). According to Zastrow (1988), successful psychotherapy succeeds because it accomplishes a change in a person's thinking from self-talk that is negative or irrational to self-talk that is more rational and positive.

According to Pedersen (2000), while we cannot exactly know clients' internal dialogue we can assume that some clients' self-talk is negative or anticounselor in orientation while other messages are procounselor and positive. The Triad Training Model simulates a forcefield of positive and negative factors from the client's viewpoint in the polarized role of the procounselor and anticounselor, who make explicit the client's positive and negative dialogue. The Model views counseling as a process of gradual oscillation between extremes of self-talk until a balance is established in which clients can reduce (negative) dependence on the problem and experiment with alternative (positive) ways of thinking, feeling, and behaving (Pedersen, 2000b).

Self-Talk and the Social Self

Pedersen (2000) subscribes to recent trends that view the self as a collective rather than monological construct (e.g., Sarbin, 1993; Hermans & Kempen, 1993). The social self is seen to be constructed via a process of inner dialogue within an individual between multicultural groups. Hermans and Kempen (1993) describe this dialogical self as a crowd of people; a diversity of subpersonalities, knowledge of which can facilitate self-growth. According to this viewpoint, awareness of dialogical self-talk, which occurs in the individual as a multicultural group, may facilitate improved awareness of multicultural identity (Pedersen & Pedersen, 1989). In terms of counselor sensitivity training, awareness that clients entertain both anticounselor and procounselor messages can enhance counselors' abilities to render effective multicultural therapy.

The Client's Internal Dialogue

Pedersen states that when two persons communicate during counseling, three simultaneously occurring conversations can be identified:

1. Both partners see and hear an exchange of verbal and nonverbal messages.
2. The counselor processes messages in his or her mind.
3. The client thinks about the alternative meanings of messages communicated by the counselor, probably debating both positive and negative interpretations of the interview as well as entertaining irrelevant information that comes to mind. The counselor is unaware of what this third conversation or internal dialogue is about (Pedersen, 1976, 1977, 1985, 1997).

Increased therapist awareness of clients' negative thoughts leads to increased client evaluation of therapists as helpful (Pedersen, 2000b). Clients frequently entertain hidden thoughts or secrets, which they do not reveal to counselors. Reasons for this may be a fear of expressing feeling, shame or embarrassment, not wanting therapists to see their limited progress, a feeling that time is insufficient, unwillingness to reveal secrets to anyone, or lack of motivation (Kelly, cited in Pedersen, 1997). Even when clients cannot articulate their negative thoughts concerning counseling, they readily admit to having them (Pedersen, 2000b). When clients hide their true reactions from therapists, especially their negative reactions, therapists' perceptions of client reactions may become distorted. The management of both quantity and quality of self-talk may be crucial in allowing therapists to maintain an appropriate focus on clients.

The anticounselor's task in the Triad Model is to articulate the client's unspoken negative reactions and therapy-resisting attitudes. The procounselor's task is to articulate positive responses that the client has toward therapy and counselor interventions. The anticounselor and procounselor make explicit the internal dialogue or self-talk of the client that a culturally encapsulated counselor may not otherwise have knowledge of.

Cognitive-behavioral interventions frequently focus on helping clients to identify faulty internal dialogues so that they may replace self-defeating internal dialogue with more constructive self-talk. Meichenbaum's work with schizophrenics and with impulsive children led him to develop Self Instructional Therapy, where clients are encouraged to monitor their self-statements or inner speech and substitute self-defeating inner talk with more adaptive and efficacious self-statements. Albert Ellis's Rational Emotive Therapy and Aaron Beck's Cognitive Therapy, arguably the most influential of the cognitive restructuring therapies, also aim at assisting clients to identify irrational self-talk and to substitute self-defeating thoughts with more adaptive beliefs. Aaron Beck has identified several faulty cognitions or "errors in logic" which are targeted for change in Cognitive Therapy. These include drawing conclusions when evidence is contradictory or lacking, exaggerating the meaning of an event, disregarding important aspects of a situation, oversimplifying events as good or bad, right or wrong, and overgeneralizing from a single event.

Many therapies utilize the notion of client internal dialogue (Pedersen, 2000b). Gestalt "deluging" helps clients explore mixed feelings and inaccurate perceptions of reality according to internalized personifications. Clients are encouraged to verbalize confusing inner thoughts in Gestalt therapy so that they can work through them, and they are encouraged to become aware and to give voice to different parts of themselves, which are seeming polarities.

Psychodramatic work has developed the alter ego concept in the training of counselors through simulations and role-plays. Janis (1982) describes an "as if" role-play in which negative messages and perspectives are explicated. In outcome psychodrama, clients project themselves into the future to articulate their worries, hopes, and unverbalised feelings.

Pedersen (2000) cites other therapies that also seek to identify and directly utilize inner process, including Schwartz's (1987) description of an "inner family" of identities within the individual. Penn and Frankfurt (1994) advocate monitoring inner conversation in family therapy in order to create new narratives. Firestone (1997a, 1997b,) has developed Voice Therapy in which patients verbalize negative thoughts toward themselves in second person "you" statements, as though they were addressing themselves. Firestone's assumption is that internal dialogue can be more punishing than actual negative events. An antiself system, comprised of accumulated negative thoughts or internalized cynical and hostile voices that attack, punish, and destroy, is targeted to help clients break with negative parental introjects. This therapy relies on the ability to conceptualize and speak to oneself as an object and to experience internalized thoughts through emotionally loaded statements.

Morin (1993) contends that self-talk can facilitate self-awareness. Engaging in dialogues with oneself and fictitious persons permits the internalization of others' perspectives. Addressing comments to oneself about oneself as others might do leads to the acquisition of self-information. Self-observation is possible only when there is a distance between the individual and any potentially observable self-aspect, as through self-talk.

Zastrow (1988) contends that the effectiveness of a variety of contemporary approaches to psychotherapy can be accounted for by the positive change that occurs when self-talk is changed. Counselor awareness of client internal dialogue is important for an understanding of how clients think about themselves, their reasons for being in therapy, and their ambivalences about engaging in therapy. A lack of sensitivity to self-talk can leave therapists ignorant about sentiments that affect clients' emotions and behaviors.

TRIAD MODEL TRAINING

Triad Training is designed to provide continuous, direct, and immediate feedback to trainees as to sources of resistance to counseling across cultures. The Triad Model assumes that the more differences there are between a counselor and a client, the more difficult it will be for a counselor to accurately anticipate client self-talk.

The anticounselor seeks to explicate the negative messages a client from another culture might be thinking but not saying while a procounselor seeks to explicate positive messages in the client's mind. An anticounselor or procounselor can participate without the other, but as noted, in more comprehensive training their combination allows both positive and negative self-talk to be heard.

Pedersen describes two Triad Training designs. The first is appropriate for approximately 10 or 12 counselors on a one-day intensive training experience. The second is appropriate for a larger group of about 30 or 40 counselors on a two-day workshop experience. Each of the designs utilizes the services of three resource persons, comprising a coached client, an anticounselor, and a procounselor. A facilitator familiar with the Model leads the training.

A trainee counselor is matched with the three resource persons for a simulated counseling interview. The resource persons come from the same background as each other but a different background to the trainee counselor. One resource person role-plays a client, another role-plays an anticounselor and a third role-plays a procounselor. The four-way conversation that ensues between the counselor, client, procounselor, and anticounselor is usually videotaped. The videotape is later reviewed by participants for debriefing and feedback.

The three resource persons should be as similar to one another as possible, for instance three persons from the same ethnic group, nationality, socio-economic group, age level, life-style, or gender role. These resource persons should be carefully selected, trained in their coached roles as client, procounselor and anticounselor, acknowledged as workshop trainers, and professionally paid. Their training involves viewing a demonstration videotape and rehearsing their roles according to directions in an accompanying manual.

THE ROLE OF THE ANTICOUNSELOR

The anticounselor triad design matches a therapist-trainee from one culture with a coached client and an anticounselor from a "contrasting" culture. The therapist seeks to build rapport with the culturally different coached client, while the anticounselor seeks to represent the problem element from the client's cultural viewpoint. The anticounselor is opposed to any successful intervention from a culturally different counselor and makes explicit the otherwise implicit resistance of culturally different clients. It is the role task of the anticounselor to try to sabotage the counseling process by emphasizing and exaggerating the negative internal messages that the client might be thinking but not saying. In deliberately being subversive and pulling in opposite directions to the counselor, the anticounselor might say or do any of the following:

1. Build on the positive things a problem has to offer, which may anchor one end of a client's ambivalence about giving the problem up.
2. Keep the interaction on a superficial level or attempt to sidetrack the counselor toward inconsequential conversation.
3. Obstruct communication by getting in-between the counselor and the client, both physically and psychologically.
4. Attempt to distract and annoy the counselor in order to draw attention away from the client, forcing the counselor to deal with defensive reactions.
5. Emphasize the importance of differences between the counselor and client to undermine the counselor's faith in his or her ability to intervene appropriately and to drive the counselor and client further apart.
6. Demand immediate, specific, and observable results from counseling.
7. Exclude the counselor by communicating privately with the client, whispering, using shared common language, or playing cultural in-jokes.
8. Find a scapegoat and ride it to deflect all blame away from the problem.
9. Attack the counselor's credibility and insist that someone more expert be called in to replace the counselor.

According to Pedersen, advantages of the anticounselor triad design are that it:

1. Forces the counselor to be aware and attuned to the client's cultural perspective.
2. Articulates negative, embarrassing, and impolite data that would otherwise remain unsaid.
3. Challenges the counselor's own defensiveness and raises his or her threshold for non-defensive responses.
4. Quickly points out the counselor's inappropriate interventions and mistakes, allowing him or her to become skilled in recovering from mistakes with increased rather than diminished rapport.
5. Forces the counselor to become skilled in focusing on the problem, since the anti-counselor constantly attempts to divert attention from it.

THE ROLE OF THE PROCOUNSELOR

Unlike the anticounselor, the procounselor attempts to facilitate effective counselor responses and to provide every opportunity for the counselor to do a better job. The procounselor identifies with the client's culture and is thus able to provide relevant cultural information and help the counselor articulate the relevant problem from the client's reference point. A skilled procounselor will help facilitate the counselor's own effectiveness without taking over the interview or distancing the counselor. The procounselor is not a cotherapist but an intermediate resource person who can guide the counselor and reinforce the counselor's more successful verbal and nonverbal strategies. The procounselor helps both the client and counselor articulate counseling as a potentially helpful process. Examples of what a procounselor may say or do include the following:

1. Restate what either the client or counselor says in a positive fashion.
2. Relate client and counselor statements to previous content and to the basic underlying problem, thus keeping things on track.
3. Offer approval or positive reinforcement for client and counselor cooperation.
4. Reinforce and emphasize important insights requiring expansion and discussion.
5. Reinforce client statements as the client becomes more cooperative in the interview.
6. Suggest alternative strategies to the counselor when necessary.

Pedersen (2000) lists the following advantages contributed by the procounselor in the simulated counseling interview:

1. When the counselor is confused or in need of support the procounselor can be consulted as a resource person.
2. The procounselor makes explicit information about the client, which might facilitate the counselor's success.
3. The procounselor provides a partner for the counselor to work with on the problem, rather than the counselor having to work alone.
4. The procounselor helps the counselor stay on track and avoid sensitive issues in ways that might increase client resistance.
5. The procounselor provides beneficial feedback to the counselor that can be used to avoid mistakes and build on successful strategies.

OPTIMAL TRAINING CONDITIONS

According to Pedersen (1977; 1983; 1985; 1988; 1997; 2000), Triad Model Training seems to work best when:

1. There is positive as well as negative feedback to the counselor.
2. The client-counselor team is highly motivated and feels strongly about the issue under discussion.
3. The anticounselor has a high degree of empathy for and acceptance by the client.
4. The anticounselor is articulate and gives direct, immediate verbal and/or nonverbal feedback to the counselor.
5. The client has not selected a real problem from his or her current situation where counseling might be appropriate. However, the discussion should be spontaneous, not scripted, and reflect actual events realistically.
6. The counselor has a chance to role-play and receive feedback three or four times in sequence.
7. The facilitator introducing the Model and leading the discussion is well acquainted with how the Model operates, the resource persons are well trained, articulate and authentic to the client's background, and the client feels free to reject an inauthentic anticounselor.
8. The simulated interview is brief (eight to ten minutes) to avoid overwhelming the counselor with information during or after the interview.
9. The interaction is videotaped to facilitate more effective debriefing.

STRENGTHS OF THE MODEL

The Triad Model provides coordinated training in cultural sensitivity through simulated role-plays in classroom-sized groups, promoting counselor growth without risk to actual clients. Counselors can make mistakes in a safe training context and receive feedback that is immediate and direct on each mistake as it occurs. The role-play interaction allows persons from different groups to train together and teach each other under controlled conditions, which minimize the dangers of parties becoming overly defended or threatened. Trainees can directly experience contact with members of a target population rather than learn about them indirectly through abstract theories.

Four specific skill areas have emerged from working with the Triad Model (Pedersen, 1977, 1978, 1983, 1985, 1997):

1. Articulating the problem from the client's cultural perspective.
2. Recognizing resistance from a culturally different client in specific rather than general terms.
3. Being less defensive in a culturally ambiguous relationship, when under attack or when receiving strong negative feedback from clients.
4. Learning recovery skills for getting out of trouble when making mistakes in counseling culturally different clients.

According to Pedersen (2000), trainees exposed to simulated role-plays should be able to generalize skills learnt to other counseling settings. Moreover, analysis of the role-play videotapes and transcripts can aid education into the impact of cultural bias in counseling contexts and the skill of separating individual differences from cultural difference.

The anticounselor and procounselor roles concretize the problem so that it becomes more than a diffuse abstraction. The role-plays explicitly provide positive and negative feedback to clarify specific sources of cooperation and resistance in the verbal and nonverbal responses of counsellees. Inappropriate counselor intervention is immediately and obviously apparent in the contest between the counselor, procounselor, and anticounselor, especially when a counselor's mistake damages the counseling relationship.

RESEARCH ON THE TRIAD MODEL

The Triad Model has been used in several hundred workshops throughout the United States to train counselors for cultural sensitivity, and has proven successful in a number of studies (e.g., Bailey, 1981; Ivey & Authier, 1978; Sue, 1979a; Wade & Bernstein, 1991). As mentioned earlier, four specific skill areas have emerged from working with the Model (Pedersen, 1977, 1978, 1983, 1985): (1) articulating the problem from the client's cultural perspective; (2) recognizing resistance from a culturally different client in specific rather than general terms; (3) being less defensive in a culturally ambiguous relationship; and (4) learning recovery skills for getting out of trouble when making mistakes in counseling culturally different clients.

Counseling students trained on the Triad Model at the University of Hawaii achieved significantly higher scores on a multiple-choice test designed to measure counselor effectiveness, had lower levels of discrepancy between real and ideal-self descriptions as counselors, and chose greater numbers of positive adjectives in describing themselves as counselors than did students who were not trained with the Model. Students also showed significant gains on Carkhuff measures of empathy, respect, and congruency as well as on seven-level Gordon scales measuring communication of affective meaning (Pedersen, 1985).

Bailey (1981) compared a traditional lecture mode of teaching intercultural skills to (1) a dyad training model, and (2) an anticounselor triad design. She found no significant differences between the Triad and the dyad training groups on effectiveness, which suggests that both approaches were equally effective but similarly superior to the traditional lecture method of intercultural training for counselors. Bailey suggested that the effectiveness of the Triad Model depends largely on how it is introduced and suggested that the Triad Model could be confusing for inexperienced trainees.

Based on his study, Sue (1979a) reported that students considered both the procounselor and the anticounselor model to contribute, in different ways, to the effectiveness of counseling with diverse ethnic groups. While students rated the anticounselor model as far superior to that of the procounselor for learning about cross-cultural counseling in the shortest period, they nevertheless felt more comfortable with the latter model, in that the anticounselor model was considered more anxiety provoking.

These findings tie in with those of Ivey & Authier (1978) who point out that naïve trainees may wilt under the pressure of the anticounselor. While suggesting Pedersen's Triad Model to be "the most powerful and direct method for crosscultural training" (p. 215), they propose that it would be most beneficial once trainees have already received training in basic micro counseling skills.

Neimeyer, Fukuyama, Bingham, Hall and Mussenden (1986) suggest that the procounselor model, in which the procounselor acts as a supportive, facilitative ally to the counselor, may be more appropriate for beginning counselors by providing them with an experience of success to alleviate their anxiety in cross-cultural interactions. The use of the more confrontative, antagonistic and subversive anticounselor agent may be better suited to the advanced student who has already developed some confidence and skill in cross-cultural interactions. Irvin and Pedersen (1995) report that there appear to be both advantages and disadvantages in experiencing either the anticounselor or procounselor first.

Wade and Bernstein (1991) found that clients assigned to experienced counselors who had received culture sensitivity training on the Triad Model rated their counselor higher on credibility and relationship measures, returned for more follow-up sessions, and expressed greater satisfaction with counseling than did clients assigned to experienced counselors who had not received the additional training. Additional studies that lend support to a growing body of findings on the utility of Triad training have been conducted by Hernandez & Kerr (1985), Chambers (1992) and Murgatroyd (1995).

The Model's Potential Utility in the Training of Family Therapists

Strous (1992) has suggested that the Triad Model and systemic family therapy appear to be compatible in many respects. This applies to their underlying aims and principles and extends to frequent similarities in their design.

In both Triad sessions as well as in family therapy practice, use is often made of videotaping, so that verbal and nonverbal messages and interactions are analyzed in a way that trainees receive corrective feedback information from peers or supervisors. Moreover, in both family therapy and Triad sessions, live on the spot supervision may be available. A family therapy team may intrude on a session when recurring nonproductive sequences entangle the therapist, or when team members feel that advice is necessary. In the Triad Model, the procounselor constantly offers advice and new directions, while the anticounselor forces the trainee to develop skills for self-disentanglement.

The use of triads, central to Pedersen's model is not unknown to systems theory and is frequently used in family therapy. Satir (1964) describes the use of triads as examples of pathogenic coalitions. She conceives of counseling as a series of negotiations in which three parties vie for control, and the therapist employs mediation and side taking to replace pathogenic relating. Zuk (1971) describes this as a "go-between" process in which the therapist catalyzes conflict in a crisis in which all parties can take an active role.

The anticounselor triad design is comparable in some ways to the "split team" or "Greek chorus" sometimes used in family therapy. The way that a split team works is that the team members criticize the family therapist in the room, acting as "a dissenting voice forming a triangle and forcing the family to take sides" (Papp, 1977). The therapist in the room may promote change, and a Greek chorus may advise against it now or against the proposed speed of change. A dissenting team offers "loyal opposition" to a therapist who is in favor of change by being skeptical, suggesting outrageous intensification of behaviors the family is already involved in, and declaring outright that the family cannot change in the way that the therapist proposes (Hoffman, 1981).

The opposition of the family therapy team to the therapist is directly comparable to the role of the anticounselor in the Triad Model, where the anticounselor deliberately opposes the trainee counselor. The split team or Greek chorus is an actual therapeutic intervention, which may result in paradoxical outcomes, while the anticounselor design is a training device. Yet, the question arises as to whether the anticounselor design is not also paradoxical in effect. The split team gives a family or client a directive that they want resisted, while an anticounselor's efforts to frustrate therapy may trigger the development of improved skills in the trainee counselor.

The procounselor triad design is comparable to cotherapy, which is frequently used by therapists in family work. As with the Triad Model, cotherapy was originally created for training purposes in order to include a trainee in a therapeutic session. In cotherapy, trainees have an opportunity to watch an expert in action and to learn a distinctive approach at close range. The trainee can also try out new approaches, assured of skilful support and rescue when trouble arises. When both therapists are experienced, cotherapy enables one of them to alternate between the relational fields of the family and the therapist. One therapist acts as a sort of lifeguard for the other therapist who may otherwise drown while exploring the sea of family patterns (Keeney, 1979; Whitaker, 1976). This is similar to the manner in which the procounselor in the Triad Model provides relevant cultural information to help the counselor articulate the relevant problem from the client's reference point. In both cotherapy and the procounselor Triad design, an attempt is made to facilitate the joining process by creating a context for adequately understanding a multiplicity of cultural and interactional patterns.

A possible anomaly that existed between earlier descriptions of the Triad Model and the evolutionary systemic approach resided in the Triad Model's reference to client resistance. Rather than viewing families as resistant, or undesirably stubborn against change, evolutionary systemic theorists prefer to see families who do not change their interactional patterns as being restrained by their belief system. The client family does not resist, say Fisch et al. (1982), it merely persists in accordance with its own structure. This led Strous (1992) to propose that focusing on the external resistance of the problem rather than on the internal resistance of clients may obviate the creation of *prima facie* objections to the Triad Model by those following an evolutionary systemic perspective.

Strong similarities exist between the manner in which Pedersen conceptualizes a problem and the writings of the Australian family therapist, Michael White (1984, 1991). Perhaps most striking is that both authors have a conceptualized understanding of problems as concrete, external manifestations that control clients. In the Triad Model, the problem is externalized and personified in the role of the anticounselor. In family therapy, Michael White attempts to effect a linguistic separation of the problem from the personal identity of the client (Tomm, 1989). For both White and Pedersen, counseling is an attempt by the counselor to seek coalition with the client against a concrete problem. Moreover, both White and Pedersen reject attempts to understand clients from the perspective of dominant ideologies. White insists on co-evolving with families in an understanding of their particular cultural stories. The emphasis is on therapy as a collaborative process, and rather than functioning as a technical wizard or behavioral engineer, the therapist acts as a conversational artist who coconstructs and coevolves as an integral part of the client system (van Zyl & Lasersohn, 1991). Both the Triad Model as well as White's conceptualization of family therapy have at their base a nonpejorative, nonjudgmental view, which represents a move away from therapist encapsulation in dominant ideologies.

The essence of both family therapy systemic thinking as well as the Triad Model is that the person-environment context must be seen as a whole. An understanding of psychological needs cannot be divorced from systemic considerations, and attempts to make psychology relevant without taking into account societal context "is dangerous and foolhardy" (Radford & Rigby, 1986, p. 16). Joining with families in a democratic and participatory way, and coevolving with their cultural and class-based perspectives, may hold the greatest promise for facilitating adaptive family responses to internal personal and external environmental events.

There are, therefore, clear similarities in the underlying precepts of systemic family therapy and the Triad Model, which suggest that the two approaches are compatible and potentially useful in promoting the cooperative endeavor between family therapists and families of diverse background in South Africa. The Triad Model and systemic family therapy have in common their use of live supervision and videotaping, their conceptualization of triads, and their focus on social and cultural context. Strong similarities exist between the anticounselor design and the Greek chorus, and the procounselor design and cotherapy. Moreover, the Triad Model and the work of Michael White have in common a conceptualization of problems as concrete, external manifestations. Both models have at their core a respect for client contexts and a nonpejorative, nonjudgmental view (Strous, 1992).

Applicability in the South African Context

Strous, Skuy and Hickson (1993) report on an investigation into family therapy supervisors' perceptions as to the potential utility of introducing Triad Model sensitivity training into family therapy training programs in South Africa. A role-play transcript of a family therapy training session using, first, a procounselor design and, second, an anticounselor design, was sent to family therapy supervisors. Results of 12 returned questionnaires reflected a significant and consistent preference for the procounselor over the anticounselor triad design, and for the anticounselor design over conventional family counseling.

The readiness of the family therapy trainers to recognize the positive value and potential effectiveness of a culturally sensitive model is seen by Strous et al. (1993) as boding well for the feasibility of its implementation. This is important given the multicultural and multiclass composition of South African society and the country's history of oppression. Ethnocentric approaches to family counseling based on dominant ideologies are often undesirable. The Triad Model offers a potentially useful adjunct to the ecosystemic family approach in that both may escape dominant culture encapsulation by remaining faithful to cultural and social contexts.

Of the three training designs considered (procounselor, anticounselor and traditional), the procounselor design was perceived as the most effective for cultural and class sensitivity training. The design is probably closest in principle to an evolutionary systemic epistemology. While the anticounselor role may not be entirely compatible with the role of the counselor as a context creator, in the procounselor design the trainee can engage in dialogical coconstruction and coevolvement with the family system. The procounselor provides relevant cultural and, hopefully, class-based information, to help trainees articulate problems from the client's reference point, in a neutral, nonjudgmental way. In both the procounselor triad model and an evolutionary systemic epistemology, the counselor or trainee counselor explores and cocreates a plethora of cultural stories, does not become encapsulated in ideologies foreign to clients, becomes an integral part of a family system, and is better able to understand and articulate the ideational context of the family. The counselor is able to acknowledge the conserving elements of both the suprasystem and internal dynamics of the family. In light of the frequently acontextual nature of South African clinical practice, it may be assumed that the Triad Model could offer useful advances on traditional family therapy training. Based on theoretical and socio-political considerations, Strous et al. (1993) conclude that the Triad Model appears to have significant potential value for the training of South African family therapists, and they recommend further research on the Model and its application. Since South African research into receptivity to the Triad Training Model has thus far only been in the field of family therapy, it is not possible at this point to make claims for individual psychotherapy. However, there is little reason to assume that the model would not be perceived as equally relevant to individual multicultural therapy training.

VARIATIONS ON THE TRIAD MODEL

Pedersen (2000) describes a number of adaptations that acknowledge the Triad Training Model as a starting point but with a variety of creative and innovative emphases and features that make them significantly different from the Triad Training Model. These innovations are:

1. The Bicultural Contextualiser (Loo, 1980a, 1980b).
2. Stereotype Reversal in Counselor Training (Jackson, 1996).
3. Cole's (1996) Proactive Approach to Reducing Prejudice.
4. The Anticlient-Proclient Model (Strous, 1997).

The Bicultural Contextualizer (BCC)

The Bicultural Contextualizer, proposed by Chalsa Loo (1980a), is a third person who places counselor and especially client messages in their appropriate context in order to clarify ethnic identity issues. The BCC is typically of the client's ethnic group and provides contextual ethnic information in order to increase the cultural sensitivity of counselors, particularly with regard to ethnic identity issues.

The BCC makes statements that provide clarification for both the counselor and client as to the counseling context. A skilled BCC allows the counselor to hear the client's thoughts as well as information that members of the client's ethnic community may have that is relevant to the counseling interview. At times, the BCC resembles a cocounselor and at times the BCC represents a coclient. Typically, the BCC functions more as a teacher or observer/participant in the interview to provide pertinent and nonevaluative ethnic information.

In the view of the present author, the BCC model seems to share some features in common with a family therapy technique proposed for use with immigrant families by Ho (1987). In this technique, a respected member of the community is selected to act as a family advocate, interpreter or "link therapist," to aid the therapist in developing and prescribing interventions. In both the BCC model and the family therapy intervention, the third person may act as a bridge between the client's worldview and social context and that of the counselor in order to facilitate accurate communication between counselors and clients from different groups.

Stereotype Reversal in Counselor Training

Margo Jackson (1996) has been engaged in researching and developing a Stereotype Reversal method at Stanford University. In this method, an anticounselor gives feedback on unintentionally biased statements by trainee counselors as if these stereotyped assumptions apply to the trainee counselors themselves, rather than to the client. Trainees thus experience the effects of racial/ethnic stereotyping first-hand. The aim is that trainees should recognize and challenge their own racially biased assumptions, including the power dynamics inherent in their own racial status; and that they should attend to individuating and stereotype-disconfirming information, including clients' strengths and assets in the social context of coping with pervasive unintentional racism. By identifying parallels between how the client is being victimized and how the counselor would feel under those same conditions, a common bond is developed between the counselor and the client across their cultural differences. In the opinion of the present author, this shoe-on-the-other-foot technique is likely to help trainees understand the stigmatizing effects of racial insensitivity. It is theoretically grounded in Ridley's (1995) perceptual schema model for developing cultural sensitivity in multicultural counseling.

Cole's Proactive Approach to Reducing Prejudice

Jim Cole (1996) has developed a training model to improve the listening skills of administrators. In this adaptation, the counselor is called a Concerned Listener, the client is called a Sharing Person, and the anticlient is called a Distracter. The Distracter questions the motives of the Concerned Listener's statements and gestures, and states the most prejudicial meaning these gestures may have. The utility of the approach is to make Triad Model Training and its associated benefits available to people not trained as professional mental health practitioners.

Anticlient-Proclient Model

While the Triad Training Model and its adaptations focus on the *client's* internal dialogue, the Anticlient-Proclient Model focuses on the *counselor's* inner dialogue. The counselor is provided with proclient statements, which he or she may draw on to facilitate effective counseling, and with anticlient statements demonstrating racism or unintentional racism, which hinder the counseling process. The Anticlient-Proclient Model is the subject of the next chapter.

SUMMARY

The Triad Model has a multicultural focus. It describes counseling as a three-way interaction between a counselor, a client, and a problem that is represented from the client's perceptual worldview. According to this conception, the counselor seeks to be helpful, the client seeks to reconcile internalized ambiguity, and the problem seeks to continue controlling the client by drawing attention to cultural differences between clients and counselors. Counselor awareness of client self-talk is viewed as important for the establishment of an effective client-counselor alliance in multicultural contexts. In order to explicate the therapy-impeding nature of client self-talk in training sessions, an anticounselor role-player seeks to personify the problem element and its associated resistance from the client's cultural viewpoint. A procounselor role-player seeks to personify therapy-facilitating elements of client self-talk. Trainees thus experience the nature of client self-talk directly, rather than learning about the nature of client resistance in multicultural settings in the abstract. A number of adaptations of the Triad Model have emerged recently. The Anticlient-Proclient Model, which will be elaborated in the next chapter, is one such innovation.

7

Hearing Counselor Self-Talk:
The Anticlient-Proclient Model

The Triad Model has potential for effective counselor sensitivity training in South Africa (Strous, Skuy, & Hickson, 1993). The anticounselor and procounselor triad designs make explicit what would be otherwise implicit inner talk of culturally diverse client groups, and are based on an appreciation of client cultural and social contexts.

The Triad Model has not, however, focused on articulating the equally important area of counselor self-talk. Minimal empirical evidence exists in the counseling literature that describes the relationship between therapists' in session cognition and therapy process variables (Nutt-Williams & Hill, 1996). As noted earlier, this may partly be due to a lack of innovative and creative means for measuring internal dialogue (Fuqua, Newman, Andersen, & Johnson, 1986; Pedersen, 2000b). There is a need to fill a crucial gap in our knowledge of counselor self-talk in multiracial counseling, but there are limited techniques for assessing this.

In order to overcome this impasse and contribute to knowledge, an extension of the Triad Model, in the form of an anticlient triad design and a proclient triad design, is proposed. The anticlient triad design that is proposed is a role personification of antagonistic or unhelpful feelings the counselor has towards counseling a racially different client. The proclient triad design that is proposed is a role personification of useful feelings and thoughts the counselor has towards counseling a racially different client.

THEORETICAL ASSUMPTIONS

The Need for Critical Awareness

As seen from the literature reviewed thus far, the mental health professions have a record of mistreating disempowered groups. A Black person in need of mental health services may be in double jeopardy because of potential shortcomings in mental health delivery in general and, in addition, the specific risk of racial discrimination within mental health systems. Many counselors occupy encapsulated positions and are unable to appreciate their clients' worldviews because of their ideologically constricted perspectives.

In contrast to counselor encapsulation, culturally effective counselors, according to Sue and Sue (1990), have the following characteristics:

1. They understand their own values and assumptions about human behavior and can recognize and accept values different from their own as legitimate.
2. They have an awareness of the generic characteristics of counseling and their relation to class and culture.
3. They act on the basis of a critical analysis and understanding of their own conditioning, that of their clients, and the sociopolitical system of which they are a part.
4. They are culturally aware, understand the basis for their worldviews and understand and accept the possible legitimacy of worldviews different from their own; and
5. They are eclectic in their counseling and able to generate the widest repertoire of microcounseling skills appropriate to the lifestyle of their individual client.

Multicultural literature advocates for increased counselor sensitivity to issues of culture. As important as this is, the promotion of cultural sensitivity without challenging racism may result in the reinforcement of racism by masking it and thereby inducing complacency (Fernando, 1986, 1988, 1991). In the context of psychiatry, Suman Fernando contends that only once a psychiatrist appreciates the social nature of racism and psychiatry's involvement in racism will that psychiatrist be ready to grapple with cultural aspects of an encounter. In Fernando's view, information concerning a patient's culture can be relatively easily obtained from the patient once barriers to communication determined by racism are broken down. How this information is used creatively and constructively may be an area of difficulty; and compromise between the practitioner and patient's explanatory models needs to be reached. However, the overcoming of cultural arrogance and its replacement with genuine concern may actually result in a quantitatively better, more beneficial rapport in an encounter involving difference than one involving similarity (Fernando, 1986, 1988, 1991).

It follows that counselors need to understand the impact of their racially informed attitudes, and assumptions that they make about their clients in racial contexts. Many counselors and therapists are, however, ill equipped to deal with racially salient material (Carter, 1995). Therapist training is generally inadequate on matters of race and racism, and therapists may be unwittingly influenced by racist ideologies that translate into discriminatory work practices (Ridley, 1995).

A difficulty in becoming aware of one's racial attitudes and racial identity is that while racial identity awareness may be conscious, issues of racial identity may also be subliminal and not readily admitted into consciousness (Helms, 1990, p. 7). The psychotherapist who is racist and/or ignorant of either his or her own conditioning or that of the client may be ineffective (Mays, 1985, p. 386). Psychotherapy, which helps patients to overcome stereotypic views of themselves, may be compromised when therapists themselves adhere to stereotypic positions (Greene, 1985, p. 389).

A critical, reflexive analysis as to how psychotherapy and counseling theory have developed within particular social and political contexts is imperative if counselors socialized within racist societies and exposed to racism within their discipline are to achieve self-awareness (Richards, 1997, xiv). Self-reflexively uncovering the socially constructed nature of social psychological explanations and showing how these explanations reproduce and maintain social power relations rather than represent neutral reality has been a key focus of critical social psychology as has been argued earlier (Henriques, Hollway, Urwin & Walkerdine, 1984; Ibanez & Iniquez, 1997; Painter & Theron, 1998; Wexler, 1983). In addition, Judy Katz (1982) submits that White people, who have been perpetrators of racist practices, need to explore their racism. White-on-White antiracism training workshops may be an appropriate way for creating positive attitudinal and behavioral change in Whites (Katz, 1982; Moore, 1973 in Katz).

Self-awareness and insight are traditional goals and themes in counseling and psychotherapy literature. Gestalt therapy has as a primary goal the attainment of self-awareness (Perls, ·1976; Simkin & Yontef, 1984). From a cognitive-behavioral perspective, Albert Ellis (1962) has identified a number of distorted ways of thinking that impair self-perspective. Psychodynamic literature has foregrounded the need for client insight, and the need for therapist self-awareness as to therapy-hindering and, in some cases, therapy- facilitating, countertransferences (Peebles-Kleiger, 1989).

Despite the emphasis in counseling literature on the need for self-awareness and insight on the part of both the client and the therapist, the potential problem in drawing attention to the conscious or unconscious racism of counselors is that such endeavors may be threatening to self-esteem and therefore resisted. As Kohut (1972) remarks, "our thought processes are taken by us as belonging to the core of our self, and we refuse to admit that we may not be in control of them" (p. 383). An immediate tendency is to deny; "primarily motivated by our shame concerning a defect in the realm of the omnipotent grandiose self" (p. 384). Kohut was writing on the subject of narcissism, but his remarks are probably applicable to many counselors who, despite the counseling ethos of self-awareness, frequently lack insight that they are behaving in racist ways (Ridley, 1995).

Personified Role-Plays

One way in which people may defend themselves against information concerning their socially unpleasant potentialities is through intellectualization. Psychologists who are frequently trained according to an academically rigorous scientist-practitioner model may be particularly prone to intellectualizing despite calls from within their own ranks for emotional growth. The problem in intellectualizing about problems is that this mechanism may allow cognitive minimization of a problem while the problem actually develops a larger-than-life impetus of its own. Nina Coltart (1995) vividly described such a process in which intellectualizing about a particular problem fuelled it in the absence of emotional working-through: "We were always talking about it, rather than it informing our talk. Gradually it became clearer how overdetermined it was, which again increased its resistant power, like the many-headed hydra, it could flourish to fight another day, even when one of its meanings could be so extensively understood that it might have lost strength through familiarity, if not through mutative interpretation" (p. 31).

Representing a problem in a personified role-play concretizes it so that it is no longer a diffuse abstraction (Pedersen, 2000b). Paul Pedersen describes a problem as concrete, complex, and constantly able to change. The concretization of the problem—defined in the Triad Model as resistance to successful therapy—explicates it as an undesirable and destructive part of the person to be addressed. Just as explicating client opposition to counselor interventions is important, so too may benefits accrue from concretizing the antagonistic attitudes of therapists in interracial therapy. The anticlient personification may explicate therapist resistance as a problem beyond intellectual abstraction with concrete ramifications.

As presented in the previous chapter, a precedent for the personification of problems is to be found in the Triad Model, Michael White's narrative family therapy approach, and a number of other therapeutic techniques. In family therapy, Michael White attempts to effect a linguistic separation of a problem from the personal identity of the client. The problem rather than the person is thus objectified. In Pedersen's Triad Model, the problem is separated from the person in such a way that it can be attacked without attacking the individual. The individual is not disassociated from the problem but recognizes the problem as a nonessential and inhibiting element of interaction with the environment.

The externalized construction of a problem reduces the likelihood of debilitating guilt and self-blame because the problem is conceptually relocated beyond the person; it is not viewed as a constituent part of the person but as an occupier, possessor, capturer, invader, and so on. (White & Epston, 1990). There is a systematic separation of problematic attributes, ideas, assumptions, beliefs, habits, attitudes and lifestyles from dominant identity (Tomm, 1989)

The personification of a part of the self as an inner saboteur is a technique also not without precedence in object-relations therapy. David Celani (1993), from a Fairbairnian perspective, describes a technique of personifying rejecting object roles in order to impress on clients, firstly, that a part of them is dominated by bad object roles and, secondly, that their whole is not all bad. A chief motivation is to improve the client's ability to form healthy attachments to others (unhindered by "antilibidinal" motivations). Celani (p. 113) writes that personifying the client's internalized rejecting object allows the therapist to discuss a toxic and unwelcome part of the self; the goal being that the individual will be able to tolerate this part of him- or herself when it emerges, accept it as a consequence of personal history, and ultimately generalize self-compassion to others. This personification of rejecting object roles that dominate the self is in some ways similar to Michael White's (1989) externalization of subjugating ideologies and to Paul Pedersen's personification of a problem as a change inhibiting force.

While Michael White and David Celani personify self-parts by getting clients to talk about them "as if" they were a person, Paul Pedersen and Gestaltist therapists instruct clients to role-play actual parts of themselves and to get these parts to converse and dialogue with each other directly. Ego-state hypnotherapy also relies on setting up conversations between different ego-states, on the assumption that multiplicity is a normal organizational principle of the human psyche, and that there can be a resolution of conflicts between the various ego-states which constitute a "family of self" within an individual (Hartman, 1993; Watkins & Watkins, 1992).

The Anticlient-Proclient Model assumes that the personification of therapist attitudes in role-plays may lead to a concretized awareness for therapists of their ambivalent attitudes towards interracial therapy. The identification and articulation of the counselor's therapy-hindering parts and therapy-facilitating parts gives voice to normally covert factors underlying interracial processes.

Tensions in the Model between Structural and Poststructural Influences

The Anticlient-Proclient Model is based on structural understandings and antistructural techniques. Socialization and cultural processes are structural in that they determine repetitive, routine, law-like behaviors and customs that many people accept unquestioningly (Appelbaum, 1998). The internalization of subtle racism, for instance, has a structural, sui generis quality in that it tends to be independent of an individual's voluntary choice or agency. The antistructural dimension of the Anticlient-Proclient Model is the personification of subtle racism and other therapy-hindering attitudes, in the hope that conscientizing therapists to therapy-hindering attitudes will permit them to exercise greater choice. The Anticlient-Proclient Model has an agency-based agenda in the sense that it tries to promote a greater degree of voluntarism on the part of counselors in examining their ideological orientation and their liberation from structural influences. The Model therefore embraces a dialectical tension between structural understandings of cultural and racial attitudes as deeply embedded and resistant to change and poststructural techniques that emphasize the need for change.

It has been argued in the above paragraph that therapy-hindering attitudes may be considered internalized and structural. The personified role-plays temporarily externalize these therapy-hindering attitudes from the personal identity of the counselor in the hope that the therapist will later choose and internalize therapy-facilitating alternatives. Thus, from the perspective of the present study, the problem may be considered internal or external, depending on the stage of training and the level of the trainee's self-awareness.

The Dialectic Opposition of Anticlient and Proclient Polarities

As noted earlier, the anticlient sentiments of White psychologists working interracially—that is, their antagonistic or unhelpful thoughts and feelings towards counseling Black patients—are likely to reflect racist ideologies rooted in colonialism, scientific racism, and notions of cultural deficit that underpin conservative psychological research and practice. Because of segregation and socialization, White psychologists may also experience anxiety in interracial counseling contexts for the reason that they have been largely removed from the psychosocial experiences that affect many of their potential clients.

Proclient sentiment, on the other hand, provides useful feelings and thoughts to counselors about counseling a racially different client. Moves in South Africa toward nonracial democracy and endeavors to democratize psychotherapy and psychological research are likely to influence the proclient positions of White psychologists. Underpinning these moves are notions of nondomination and equality, which dovetail with an ideology of human rights.

The Anticlient-Proclient Model polarizes these two positions and concretizes them by getting counselors to role-play anticlient and proclient parts of themselves. This creates dialogical possibilities for improved self-awareness as to the influence of racial attitudes in interracial counseling contexts and may permit counselor's greater choices in how to respond effectively in interracial settings. South African and many other therapists have been exposed to the competing values of racism, counseling theory, and moves toward democratization. In order to depict the discrepancy between elements to which therapists have been exposed, the Anticlient-Proclient Model conceptualizes the anticlient position and the proclient position as standing in dialectical opposition to each other. The anticlient and proclient personifications thus represent polarized positions and the therapist or counselor is acknowledged as having polarized sides or parts to him- or herself, resulting in ambivalent attitudes.

The interplay of opposite characters is characteristic of narrative approaches (Hermans & Kempen, 1993, p. 163). Narrative approaches to psychotherapy have decentralized the self and recognized a multiplicity of "I" positions (Sarbin, 1993), each having their own voice and stories to tell. In this perspective, "The I moves, in an imaginal landscape, from one position to another in such a way that dialogical relationships in a multivoiced self become possible" (Hermans & Kempen, p. xxi). This decentralized multiplicity of divergent and even opposite characters is in line with the postmodern notion of the self as being constituted by a multiplicity of parts (Bakker, 1996).

Cognitive behavioral accounts similarly conceive of inner speech—the conscious dialogues we hold with ourselves (Berk, 1994)—as a dialogue between two polarized sides of the person, such as rational versus irrational beliefs, or negative versus positive attributes. A dialectic approach, which permits one to flip-flop between different perspectives, holds open the possibility of increased appreciation for the dynamic relationships that exist between different levels of systemic experience (Combrink-Graham, 1987). Ongoing dialogical relationship between mind and meaning systems allows for vibrant changes through new contributions and/or gradual deletion of old patterns (Shweder, 1990).

From a Gestaltist perspective, insight may result when one grasps the unity of disparate elements in a field. Such awareness, accompanied by "owning," promotes the process of knowing one's control over, choice of, and responsibility for one's behavior and feelings (Simkin & Yontef, 1984, p. 290).

The relationship between the anticlient and proclient roles is dialectic. As is characteristic of other dialectical relationships, "they are contradictory and necessarily interrelated. The threads are knotted together ... such that they only take the tangled shape they do because they exist together, around each other. They exist as a 'unity of opposites,' and are played out ... in a dynamic 'strategy of tension'" (Parker, 1999, p. 4).

Rowan & Cooper (1999) note that a number of self-pluralistic approaches propose that an individual can be conceptualized as a plurality of qualitatively distinct selves as well as a one: an interpenetrative, dialogical constellation of subselves (Martindale, 1980; Shapiro, 1976), subpersonalities (Assagiol, 1965; Rowan, 1990; Stone and Winkelman, 1989), ego states (Berne, 1961; Watkins and Watkins, 1979-80), voices (Hermans et al., 1993), parts (Schwartz, 1995), roles (Landy, 1993), alter egos (Grotstein, 1997), potentials (Mahrer, 1996), or selves and others (Shotter, 1997).

Where there is a lack of communication, where selves disown each other or where one self dominates to the exclusion of all others, then the result tends toward a cacophony of monologues—a discordant wail which will always be less than the sum of the individual parts. But where selves talk to selves, where there is an acceptance and understanding between the different voices and an appreciation of diversity and difference, then there is the potential for working together and cooperation—an interwoven harmony of voices which may transcend the sum of the parts alone. (Rowan & Cooper, 1999, p. 8)

The functionality of self-plurality is fundamentally related to the level of dialogue between the different selves (Rowan & Cooper, 1999). The Anticlient-Proclient Model is based on the premise that counselors need to hear the competing inputs of two specific sides of themselves; one that is receptive to or pro- interracial therapy and the other that is negative toward it. The anticlient and proclient personifications literally put words in the mouth of a counselor in order to concretely articulate the dialectic opposition and dialogical interaction of their positions

THE ANTICLIENT ROLE

Internal self-talk has been described by Mackay and Fanning (1994) as: "a voice-over commentary on what you see on the screen in your head. Your self-talk can contain the destructive comments of your internal pathological critic, or your healthy refutations of the critic. The voice-over interprets and can distort what you see. Sometimes you are aware of the voiceover, but often you are not" (1994, p. 137).

What might the voice-over of the therapist be when articulating an anticlient position? It is likely that in expressing feelings that are racially insensitive, anticlient opinions will be antithetical to the principles of multicultural psychology, client empowerment, social advocacy and human rights. The anticlient position is likely to be founded in conservative social and political attitudes, racism, deprecatory client assessment and denigrative self-evaluation of the counselor's own training and skills to work interracially. More specifically, some things the anticlient position may influence a counselor to say or do could include the following:

1. Provide reasons for the counselor to maintain distance and defensiveness in the interview.
2. Emphasize cultural, racial and language differences between the counselor and client in a negative way, and convey a sense of futility in the communication.
3. Capitalize on the counselor's conflicts that distort perceptions and contaminate therapy.
4. Build on the more positive things a problem offers in comparison to counselor interventions.
5. Capitalize on the complications of the problem.
6. Inform the counselor to keep interventions superficial, obscure and ineffectual.
7. Give reasons for the counselor to overextend and move too rapidly.
8. Influence the counselor to antagonize clients subtly or directly.
9. Sidetrack the counselor by focusing on his or her personal issues that are triggered by the therapy.
10. Supply misinformation as to how client and counselor racial identity statuses interact.
11. Capitalize on often held stereotypes about multiracial therapy that are unquestionably assumed true in most cases. Inferences drawn from various literatures on cross-cultural counseling, interracial therapy and class-based analyses may be exaggerated and may lead to counselors feeling demotivated about their ability to successfully render appropriate services in interracial contexts. The following stereotypes (which are raised in the literature or which have implications resonant with the present researcher's own experiences) may emerge:

- Blacks are unresponsive to psychotherapy.
- Whites are inadequately equipped to counsel Blacks.
- White racism interferes with therapeutic processes.

The list that follows comprises a fairly inclusive inventory of constructs noted as problematic in cross-racial therapeutic work. Counselors who are ideologically encapsulated may explicitly verbalize some of the following notions that could undermine faith in interracial therapy:

Concepts of psychotherapy are alien to the thinking of Blacks.
Blacks are unresponsive to long-term therapy and individualized psychotherapeutic approaches.
Blacks would rather consult indigenous faith healers.
Blacks, or their version of events, cannot be trusted.
Blacks are violent.
Blacks are AntiWhite.
Blacks are cognitively inferior to Whites.
Blacks have a fundamentally different view of time to counselors.
Black worldviews and Euro-American psychotherapies cannot be reconciled.
Blacks view counseling as a mystifying process, are reluctant to self-disclose, and will show a paranoid mistrust of White counselors.
Blacks are unable to use therapy usefully.
Blacks desire professionally provided solutions rather than self-insight. Blacks are action-orientated and concrete thinkers. This contradicts therapeutic endeavors, which rely on abstract thinking.
Blacks expect counselors to behave authoritatively, like doctors.
The material concerns of Blacks negate their interest in matters psychological.
The external realities of Black life are so compromising to mental health that there is little point in attempting to be empathically sensitive to their inner worlds.
Few Blacks can afford therapy.
White counselors cannot appreciate Black nonverbal cues and customs.
White counselors separated from the daily encounters of Black existence cannot form any meaningful understanding of the mind and behavior of Blacks.
Something about the emotional life of Blacks is mysterious and unknowable to Whites.
Western psychological approaches cannot accommodate the spiritual views of Blacks.
First World therapy should not be used with Third World clients.
Eurocentric strategies have nothing to offer Black clients.
Language differences render senseless the oral communications of White therapists.
Medication is a cheaper and more affordable intervention than multiracial counseling.
(Abdi, 1975; Anonymous, 1986; Berger & Lazarus, 1987; Dawes, 1986; Gillis, Koch & Joyi; 1989; Hayes, 1986; Hickson & Kriegler, 1996; Littlewood & Lipsedge, 1997; Moosa, 1992; Sue & Sue, 1977; L. Swartz, 1991; Thomas & Sillen, 1972; Turton, 1986).

These anticlient statements are based on abstractions of the reviewed literature as well as additional readings resonant with the researcher's personal experiences or observations of interracial therapy. Local and international literature on mental health and racism, transference and countertransference, counselor encapsulation, racial identity, and Pedersen's Triad Model influenced the identification of the above anticlient statements. The researcher is also aware of the following personal factors that influenced his selection and formulation of the anticlient statements:

1. Insecurity concerning whether therapy training equips counselors to meet the needs of Black clients;
2. Awareness that a lack of understanding of Black languages and idiomatic expression curtails effective counseling;
3. A conception that the material needs of the underprivileged Black community are so enormous that working on an emotional level should be secondary to the amelioration of material needs;
4. Processes of socialization in a racist and intolerant society can inadvertently influence White counselors' to stereotype Black clients; and
5. Exposure to literature and training that focus on the difficulties of interracial therapy may improve awareness to guard against countertherapeutic practices, but may also be demotivating.

THE PROCLIENT ROLE

In stating the counselor's therapy-facilitating thoughts and feelings, the proclient position is likely to reveal the advantages of cultural, class and racial sensitivity in therapy; to show allegiance to the principles of multicultural and community psychology, such as client empowerment and democratic power sharing; and to convey appreciation for human rights. More specifically, the proclient could:

1. Use the counselor's feelings to help the counselor understand the client's hopes, values, and predicaments.
2. Alert the counselor that his or her responses possibly replicate how other people perceive the client and can therefore provide useful information.
3. Inform the counselor of his or her own responses to a client's behavior that other people in the client's context deem to be socially unacceptable.
4. Explicitly verbalize empathic reactions that the counselor feels in relation to the client.
5. Offer approval to the counselor about his or her counseling endeavors, and provide objective and beneficial feedback to the counselor about his or her role in the therapy process.
6. Elucidate the advantages of joining with clients in a phenomenological understanding of their worldview.
7. Encourage counselors by expressing faith in their ability to join with clients from diverse groups.
8. Assist the counselor in overcoming his or her own defensiveness.
9. Help the counselor to tackle racially salient issues in a sensitive manner.
10. Supply intuitive as well as informed feedback as to how different levels of racial identity between clients and counselors may be optimally used to improve therapeutic rapport.

These proclient interventions are antithetical to the therapy-hindering interventions (anticlient statements) that were formulated. The proclient formulations were influenced by abstractions from the literature that are concordant with the researcher's personal sympathies; notably:

1. A phenomenological concern based on caring, and a desire to help people through suffering and misery;
2. Awareness of the historical misrepresentation of Blacks and the supposed worldview of Black clients; and
3. A commitment to human rights.

(e.g., Carter, 1995; Essed, 1991; Pagels, 1979; Pedersen, 1997; Prilletensky, 1997; Richards, 1997; Rogers, 1967; van der Vyfer, 1976; van Dijk, 1993).

In addition to the anticlient and proclient verbalizations listed above, the anticlient and proclient could also use nonverbal behaviors to reveal like or dislike for the client, the client's problems, emotions or behaviors. This would give added, visual, impact to the explication of frequently hidden counselor sentiment concerning clients.

THE TRAINEE COUNSELOR

The task of the trainee counselor in the Anticlient-Proclient Model is to articulate his or her attitudes toward interracial therapy and to engage in dialogue with the anticounselor and the procounselor. The counselor might:

1. Agree with either the anticlient or the proclient and increase his or her behaviors in accordance with either or both of their observations or suggestions.
2. Disagree with either the anticlient or the proclient and decrease his or her behaviors in reaction to either or both of their prescriptions or observations.
3. State ambivalence concerning the competing suggestions or demands of the anticlient and the proclient.

The shifting positions and behaviors of the trainee counselor during the interview would be indicative of the therapy-hindering or therapy-facilitating influences of the anticlient or proclient respectively.

THE CLIENT ROLE

As in the Triad Model, the person role-playing the client in Anticlient-Proclient training could be drawn from a different social or racial group to the counselor. However, anticlient attacks against the client, albeit for training purposes, could result in misgivings, even on an unconscious level. Thus, it may be judged better, at least initially, for the client's position to be articulated in one of the following ways:

1. A role-player from the counselor's own social group could try to approximate what a client from a different group might say or do.
2. The client's problem or dynamics could be presented on videotape or in script form, and the counselor, anticlient and proclient could respond as to what their positions are likely to be without interacting directly with a client role-player.
3. Articulations by the anticlient and the proclient could be filtered through an earpiece to the trainee counselor and in this way be kept out of earshot of the person role-playing the client. This would necessitate a change in the counselor's role in that the trainee counselor would respond aloud only to the client, not to the anticlient or proclient who would be seated behind a one-way mirror.
4. The anticlient and the proclient may respond to the client-counselor interaction from behind a one-way mirror, out of earshot of both the client and the counselor, but in the presence of an observing team. The observing team and/or the anticlient and proclient could later inform the counselor as to their talk during the role-play. Many institutions that train therapists are well equipped with one-way mirrors and intercom links.

ADVANTAGES OF AN ANTICLIENT-PROCLIENT MODEL

A new proclient-anticlient triad design should prove conceptually useful in assessing data as to counselor motivations, intentions and interactions in cross-racial settings.

1. A focus on the counselor's therapy-facilitating and therapy-impeding self-talk is in line with a new paradigm in psychology which views the "dialogical self" as a multicultural self, constructed and reconstructed from encounters with others and reciprocal influences of a cultural society (Hermans & Kempen, 1993; Pedersen, 2000b; Sarbin, 1993).
2. The resolutions of competing proclient and anticlient self-messages can be explored. In his discussion of the Triad Model, Pedersen draws attention to forcefield analyses. A forcefield is the social-psychological field that immediately surrounds a decision or action, including an individual's perception of forces that compel or restrain alternative actions (Lewin, 1969). Comparisons between proclient-anticlient negotiations, the notion of multivoiced selves in the complex area of moral conflict (Sarbin, 1993), and the notion of ego status resolutions in racial identity theory (Helms, 1990) could hold interesting possibilities.
3. Analysis of Anticlient-Proclient negotiations would acknowledge that counselor attitudes and countertransference issues contain both positive and negative therapy influences, and their outcome is dependent on the power influence of both. This is compatible with countertransference as hindrance as well as with countertransference as facilitator models (Peebles Kleiger, 1989). Considering both positive and negative dimensions of self-talk simultaneously "and framing the polarity idea in terms of the balance between the opposing roles represents an integrative step with potential heuristic value" (Swartz & Garamoni cited by Pedersen, 2000b, pp. 6465).
4. The Triad Model is theoretically consistent with the social psychology literature of counseling as a coalition formation process (Pedersen, 2000b). In the case of the Proclient-Anticlient Model, the influence of the therapy-hindering and the therapy-facilitating inner-talk of counselors could be incorporated into coalition analysis formulations.
5. Use of the Triad Model and its proposed extension need not be exclusive to any school of psychology. The Triad Model draws on a number of psychological traditions, including perspectives from psychodynamic therapy, cognitive-behavior therapy, narrative approaches, Gestalt psychology, and psychodrama. The Triad Model is not bound to any of these paradigms but can accommodate all of them. The Triad Model offers a theoretical interface between social psychology and counseling psychology (Pedersen, 2000b) and is compatible with many ideals and goals of community psychology, multiracial counseling, integrative analyses of prejudice, and theories of social and racial identity.
6. An opportunity could be provided for role-playing or discussing initial incidents in cross-cultural and cross-racial counseling under controlled conditions.
7. Cultural problems and racial identity issues are made specific rather than abstract.
8. Externalizing and personifying countertransference issues in the role of an anticlient could ameliorate counselor defensiveness or the desire of therapists not to express politically incorrect attitudes. An Anticlient-Proclient Model could prove a nonjudgmental base for investigating countertransference issues. In a manner similar to that used in the systemic narrative therapy of Michael White (1984, 1986a, 1986b, 1991; White & Epston, 1990), self-defeating ideologies could be linguistically separated from one's personal identity.
9. Perceptions of discontinuity between the role-played and the role-player may permit increased "leakage" of the self (Yardley, 1995) for later analysis.

10. The counselor could become increasingly aware of his or her unspoken self-talk as it influences counseling.
11. Counselor self-talk could be recorded on videotape or as a transcript and analyzed. A careful analysis of the typescripts could identify counseling skills appropriate or inappropriate to different multiracial counseling contexts.
12. In contradiction to the Triad Model, the Anticlient-Proclient design requires no coached team apart from the trainee therapists themselves. This has advantages in terms of time, finances and logistics.

POSSIBILITIES FOR IMPLEMENTING THE MODEL

A wide variety of training situations and role-play combinations are possible. The following is an exhaustive list of single, dyadic, and triadic role-play combinations:

1. Single role-play personifications:
   The anticlient alone
   The proclient alone
2. Dyads:
   Anticlient-client
   Proclient-client
   Anticlient-Proclient
   Anticounselor-anticlient
   Procounselor-anticlient
   Counselor-anticlient
   Counselor-proclient.
3. Triads:
   Anticlient-client-proclient
   Anticlient-client-anticounselor
   Anticlient-client-procounselor
   Anticlient-counselor-proclient
   Anticlient-counselor-anticounselor
   Anticlient-counselor-procounselor
   Proclient-client-anticounselor
   Proclient-client-procounselor
   Procounselor-counselor-proclient
   Procounselor-counselor-anticounselor
   Proclient-counselor-procounselor.

Figure 2 illustrates a multitude of lines of potential communication. Each line, joined at the center with another line or set of lines, depicts that each participant may be linked with any other participant(s) in a plethora of role-play combinations. The largest possible combination would be one of client, counselor, anticlient, proclient, anticounselor and procounselor. Combinations of four or five role-players are also possible, as are triads, dyads and single role-play personifications.

Figure 2
Lines of Interactional Communication when Triad Model and Anticlient-Proclient Elements Are Combined

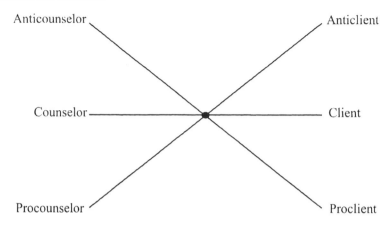

The greater the number of ideologically authoritative and independent characters that are role-played, the more the exercise may provide a polyphony of voices (Bakhtin, 1973), accompanying and opposing each other in dialogical relation, and potentially leading to the emergence of meanings that are not available at any one of the given positions alone (Hermans & Kempen, 1993). In the interests of coherence and simplicity, it will be necessary to choose judiciously from the available combinations for purposes of racial sensitivity training.

Some of the combinations discussed could provide ethical dilemmas. When an anticlient attacks in the presence of a client, anticounselor, or procounselor, the anticlient is attacking a member of another cultural or racial group. The goal is sensitivity to culture and nonracism, but the means will require consideration. One way of dealing with the dilemma of not affronting members of other racial or cultural groups, even for training purposes, may be for a team behind a one-way mirror to hear anticlient messages out of earshot of the other role-players. This, however, raises issues of elitism and exclusion. It could also lessen the impact of training.

Paul Pedersen (personal communication) has suggested that there could be a more reduced risk in having persons take on the anti or pro role during brief (five to eight minute) role-played interviews than might be imagined, especially when there is clear and careful definition of roles beforehand and debriefing. According to Pederson (personal communication), it is expected that both the anti and the pro will exaggerate messages in a kind of tug-of-war between the anti and pro messages the client might be thinking. Only by monitoring the reaction of the client will the counselor trainee be able to evaluate the degree of accuracy in the anti and pro messages. If the counselor becomes his or her own procounselor or anticounselor, there is a danger of role diffusion. By having the pro and anti voices simultaneous with the role-played interview (multiple simultaneous conversations), the normal screening that protects us from hearing our own possibly hidden thoughts breaks down. The trainee might then gain insight into unconscious thoughts he or she has but has avoided articulating.

Because role-plays offer an opportunity to deliberately construct particular therapy processes and engage people in roles that would normally be vigorously hidden (Yardley, 1995), it is important to explicitly contract with participants over expected levels of personal disclosure. It is also important that participants be deroled and debriefed following their role-play of personified parts.

Finally, the Anticlient-Proclient Model has been designed with the specific purpose of explicating counselors' attitudes towards interracial therapy. The model could, however, be used for helping counselors and therapists to gain insight in any counseling context in which counselors experience ambivalent thoughts or feelings towards clients.

SUMMARY

The effectiveness of interracial therapy may be compromised because many counselors occupy encapsulated positions, unaware of their ideologically constricted perspectives. Counselors may also fail to appreciate the racially sensitive nature of their competing perspectives. Representing these therapy-hindering and therapy-facilitating elements in personified role-plays seems to hold promise for helping counselors to move beyond intellectualized abstraction concerning interracial therapy, and could help to facilitate the development of a more critically informed self-awareness for counselors. An Anticlient-Proclient triad design has been proposed, therefore, in order to explicate both positive and negative counselor self-talk in interracial therapy. The anticlient triad design comprises a role personification of antagonistic or unhelpful feelings that a counselor harbors towards counseling a racially different client, while the proclient design articulates a counselor's positive thoughts and feelings towards interracial therapy. The Anticlient-Proclient triad design has only been studied conceptually, but is, arguably, potentially useful in cultural and racial sensitivity training workshops.

8

Difference and Interplay between Anticlient and Proclient Positions: Initial Research Findings

According to research conducted at the University of the Witwatersrand, Johannesburg (Strous, 2001; Strous & Eagle, in process), the anticlient and proclient positions can be differentiated in terms of polarized characteristics. However, counselor behavior is not fixed in one particular position. Counselors tend to weigh up the pros and cons of anticlient and proclient claims and intermittently flip-flop between their attendant and opposing dynamics.

INITIAL RESEARCH

The first investigation into the Anticlient-Proclient Model (Strous, 2001) aimed to investigate how counselors' negative attitudes to interracial counseling reflect ideologies pertaining to racism in South Africa and South African psychology, how their positive attitudes reflect positions related to racial sensitivity, and how these competing positions are negotiated when counselors reflect on them. In order to explore these aims, psychologists in private practice were interviewed as to:

1. their inner dialogue that was therapy-facilitating,
2. their inner dialogue that was therapy-hindering, and
3. the likely resolution and influence of their therapy-facilitating and therapy impeding inner dialogue(s).

During the course of each interview, a structured exercise based on the Anticlient-Proclient Model was introduced. Participants were asked to adopt the personae, alternatively, of their therapy-hindering (anticlient) side and their therapy-facilitating (proclient) side. The researcher interviewed these different personas. The participants were then asked to alternate between their therapy-hindering and therapy-facilitating voices, in order to get these parts to dialogue with each other.

The role personification of therapy-hindering and therapy-facilitating notions held by counselors seemed to have facilitated increased self-disclosure on the sensitive topic of racial attitudes through, *inter alia*:

1. The fictional separation of the participants and the role-play situation, which may have permitted greater "leakage" of self.

2. The linguistic separation of the counselor from his or her therapy-hindering positions (personified in the anticlient role), which may have protected counselor self-esteem.
3. Tracking of the counselors' proclient positions, which provided an alternate focus to only focusing on anticlient perspectives

The interviews were recorded verbatim. Analysis of the typescripts was then conducted using a grounded theory approach that included deconstructive elements (Charmaz, 1995; Layder, 1993; Pidgeon, 1996; Pidgeon and Henwood, 1996).

The anticlient sentiments of White psychologists working interracially—that is, their antagonistic or unhelpful thoughts and feelings toward counseling Black patients—were found to be influenced largely by Whitecentric notions of Blacks as different and inferior. It was also found that White psychologists could experience anxiety and feelings of being overwhelmed in interracial counseling contexts. The proclient sentiments of White psychologists, on the other hand, were found to be informed by notions of racial sensitivity, nondomination, equality, consultative participation, flexibility, and motivation to be as effective as possible in the context of a healing relationship (Strous & Eagle, in process).

An important finding of the study was that therapists' attitudes toward interracial therapy might fluctuate as therapists entertain the competing truth claims of anticlient and proclient perspectives. Figure 3 depicts a model of therapist ambivalence with reference to the iterative links between anticlient and proclient conceptualizations and their respective outcomes. This diagrammatic representation juxtaposes the contradictory perspectives and dynamics of the competing anticlient and proclient positions, and provides a framework for their comparison.

ANTICLIENT AND PROCLIENT POSITIONAL DIFFERENCES

Whitecentricism Versus "Equality in Diversity"

A fundamental difference between the anticlient and the proclient positions in interracial therapy is that the anticlient position is characterized by Whitecentricism whereas the proclient position recognizes equality in diversity. Whitecentricism is the ideal and practice whereby interests and perspectives of the White group are taken as central and normative, and Black interests and perspectives are marginalized (Essed, 1991). White therapists, when acting from an anticlient perspective, frequently define reality according to their own worldviews and take for granted that their clients must accommodate to their way of seeing things. This confirms suggestions in the literature that White clinicians, schooled, socialized, and trained in ways that cocooned them from multicultural, socio-economic, and racial realities, are likely to have a truncated appreciation of factors informing the worldviews of many Black clients. In contradiction to this limitation of perspective, therapists operating from a proclient perspective are mindful not to impose dominant White values on Black clients. Proclient ideals of nonracism and cultural sensitivity stand in contraposition to the anticlient perspective. The proclient attempt to substitute potentially subjugating definitions of racial identity with more open-minded and flexible constructs affirms the notion of equality in diversity.

Figure 3
The Anticlient-Proclient Model of Therapist Ambivalence

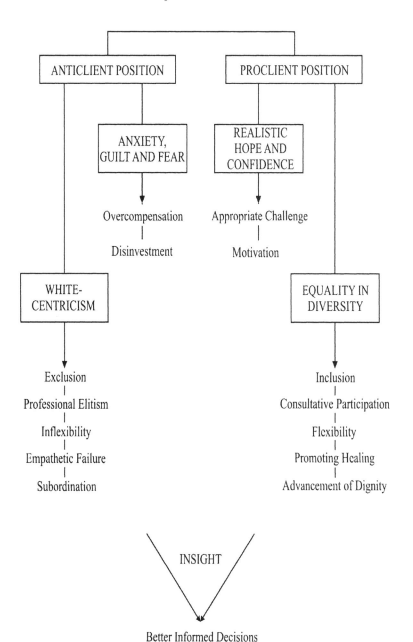

Theorists within the field of subtle racism (e.g., Crosby, Bromley & Saxe, 1980; McConahay, Kinder & Sears, 1981) suggest that there has been a shift from overt, explicit expressions of racist beliefs to subtler, symbolic forms of racism. The study indicated that White therapists might perpetuate features of modern racism that construct other cultures as disadvantaged, by problematizing Black culture as deviating from preferred, Western standards of psychological health. From an anticlient perspective, deviations from White values and behavioral norms were frequently viewed as pathological. While such constructions could have appeared objective and even sympathetic from a noncritical perspective, closer scrutiny revealed that there was a lack of interrogation of the assumptions underlying the interviewees' constructs and an implicit patronization. Within the interviews, there were allusions to Black culture as overly reliant on violence to solve conflict, there were implications that Black society was perceived as developmentally retarded with regard to gender equality, and there were constructions of Black family life and parenting as substandard. Inadequately developed standards of morality were suggested in allusions to Blacks as unduly entitled, backed up in one case with reference to a "national level narcissistic injury." The term "national level narcissistic injury," initially used to refer to Nazi Germany as a threat to Western society (Kohut, 1972), was used in this instance by one of the participants who cautioned that Blacks can be vengeful when they do not get what they want. Constructions of Blacks as irrational, with an underdeveloped sense of morality, underpinned a number of the interviews. The interviews further revealed assumptions by some of the participants that Black clients would be hostile toward White therapists or unable to trust helpers outside of their own communities. These assumptions contributed to a deficit-oriented view of Black culture by raising questions as to Black clients' abilities to participate in therapeutic systems based on Western norms. These assumptions also appeared to place the responsibility for their own pathology, damage, and inability to access psychotherapy on Black people themselves. Such constructions omitted the contextualization of observed patterns of Black behavior within relations of racial dominance and tended to essentialize features of Black culture. In keeping with modern forms of racism, such constructions were generally characterized by deficit oriented discourses rather than more crude forms of racism. Subtle beliefs and assertions such as these may be more difficult to interrogate as racist than is crude racism, and from this perspective the anticlient design and associated role-playing appeared particularly useful in encouraging therapists to examine and question these assumptions.

In contraposition to the anticlient position, which affirms the superiority of White culture, the proclient position values people from other cultural and racial groups and recognizes strengths in their different backgrounds. The proclient perspective recognizes that negative group stereotyping may lead to the denial of individual uniqueness. It is important from a proclient perspective to understand both differences and similarities between races, without amplifying these differences in a negative evaluation of any racial group.

The interviews revealed that from a proclient perspective, and in the South African context in particular, there are risks involved in relating to Blacks on the assumption that their worldview differs from the worldview of Whites and on the assumption that cultural diversity dominates all other considerations. While the therapists operating from a proclient position displayed an awareness of indigenous resources and an acceptance of the need to learn about other cultures and races, many of them nevertheless voiced caution that clients should not be pigeonholed according to racial labels. The implication of this is that Black clients wishing to engage in Western-style psychotherapies should not be excluded from doing so. Although the simultaneous recognition of diversity and universals is a difficult tension to embrace, the proclient role-play allowed therapists to entertain such ambiguity more openly than did the ideological closure implicit in the anticlient position.

Inclusion Versus Exclusion

The objectification and problematization of Blacks in dominant ideology serves to legitimize their exclusion from White society (Essed, 1991). The study revealed that in the field of psychotherapy, counselors ensconced in anticlient traditions were often reluctant to engage with Black clients with the same amount of effort that they reserved for White clientele. This was voiced on the basis that there was no time to educate "unsophisticated" Blacks who were not conversant with therapeutic traditions, or on the basis that Eurocentric techniques might be inapplicable to Blacks. Black clients would therefore be excluded from the full benefits that psychotherapy might afford. This would constitute a form of institutional racism. Racism may be defined as any behavior or pattern of behavior that tends to systematically deny access to opportunities or privileges to members of one racial group while perpetuating access to opportunities and privileges to members of another racial group (Ridley, 1989). An exclusionary dimension of anticlient position outcomes could perpetuate the inferiority of mental health services traditionally provided to Black patients and the underrepresentation of Black mental health practitioners.

In contradiction to the anticlient perspective, the proclient position is compatible with human rights provisions for full and inclusionary group participation. A fundamental aspect of the proclient position that was revealed through the interviews was a willingness to share professional resources with members of disempowered groups. As opposed to exclusionary practices of racism, therapists operating from a proclient position readily embraced interracial therapy as desirable. They endorsed a view of therapy as being as broad and inclusive as possible and they voiced willingness to engage with Black patients. This applied to training more Black counselors and ensuring the contextual appropriateness of counseling techniques. It could be theoretically argued, especially in the South African context, that commitment to interracial therapy would also be well served by material initiatives such as making services accessible in terms of locale and payment.

Professional Elitism Versus Consultative Participation

The proclient position endorses a view of active client engagement in the therapeutic process in a spirit of participative consultation with counselors. Partnership between clients and counselors was valued by a number of the participants over professional elitism and the centralization of expert power. The term "consultative participation" implies a dual process:

1. commitment to inclusionary principles, in which professional resources are available to people from all groups; and

2.   checking out of therapeutic perceptions, plans, and goals with clients, in order to avoid the imposition of counselor perspectives on clients who may hold different points of view.

Whereas proclient allegiance to power sharing is signaled through commitment to actively involving clients in problem identification, goal setting and decision making, the anticlient position is characterized by the autocratic imposition of counselor-generated formulations and interventions. In an anticlient role, the counselor might represent a doctor displaying superior medical knowledge, or could be thought of in Hoffman's terms (1981) as a bullfighter who pushes and pulls patients around to get them to do what he or she wishes. On the other hand, proclient themes of equality and diversity, and the affirmation of group distinctiveness and value, are coupled with the expression of a need to limit professional authority.

In moving toward consensual cooperation and more equal distributions of power in therapy, the proclient position does not appeal for abandonment of professional responsibility. Counselors operating from a proclient role were mindful of the need to value client perceptions, goals, and rights to self-determination, without disempowering themselves through an abdication of their role as effective helpers or a negation of their ability to influence through the power of suggestion. While some of the counselors remained concerned that confronting clients could undermine democratic and nonjudgmental initiatives through the excessive use of power, they were aware at the same time that nonuse of appropriate confrontation could also lead to less effective therapy.

The proclient recognition of the need to allow clients equal participation and the focus on limiting authoritarianism and elitism in psychology is in keeping with democratic principles. The study substantiated observations that notions of participative consultation and collaborative action, and anticlient notions of elitism and authority, are dichotomous processes. However, there appears to be a need to distinguish more accurately between proclient exercises of power that are therapeutically beneficial and anticlient autocracy that invalidates client perceptions.

Inflexibility Versus Flexibility

Consistent with the literature on counselor sensitivity (e.g., Sue 1981; Pedersen, 1997; Ridley, 1995), the proclient position advocates for flexible case formulations and interventions in different cultural and/or racial contexts. For instance, therapists operating from a proclient position expressed a need to move from White, Westernized, and Eurocentric practices toward integrated therapies that match the worldviews of clients and accommodate indigenous diagnostic and healing practices where appropriate. The proclient perspective on flexibility requires that therapists technically apply their knowledge and skills in a manner that is accommodating of local perspectives and that is mindful of the views of traditionally oppressed groups. This contradicts anticlient processes, in which therapists inflexibly adopt etic approaches to mental health interventions regardless of social contexts.

The anticlient position is characterized by inflexibility on the part of encapsulated counselors, who dogmatically adhere to what Pedersen (1976, 1997) has called "technique-oriented notions of universal truth." The anticlient position reflects uniracial and unicultural perspectives as well as counselor expectations that clients should adjust to professional perspectives on mental health. In opposition to this, the proclient position advocates, as one participant put it, that: "there is no one value system that is correct; there is no one worldview that is correct; there is no one intervention that is correct."

Empathic Failure Versus the Promotion of Healing

The anticlient position frequently results in empathic failure on the part of counselors. Empathy is a form of human communication that involves both listening and understanding *and* the communication of that understanding to clients (Egan, 1986, pp. 8687). The research findings supported suggestions that White therapists influenced by racially pejorative perspectives may relate to Black people through a cultural lens or in terms of racial categories, such that they neither see nor treat an individual (Kagan, 1964), and that racially stereotyped assumptions and prescriptions can negate the individual uniqueness and worth of clients (Jones & Seagull, 1977). A number of the participating psychologists referred to negative discrimination as having dehumanizing consequences. For instance, exposure to apartheid ideology might influence counselors to be primarily concerned with classifying people according to cultural categories rather than recognizing their essential personhood. This implies that over focusing on cultural classification can result in the intellectual reification of individuals that denies their humanity.

Participants suggested that because of their encapsulation they might experience greater difficulty in bonding with Black clients and in exploring pertinent issues than they would with White clients. A central finding of the study was that White therapists' discomfort, fear, guilt, and guardedness around Blacks might impede both their empathy and spontaneity in interracial contexts. These findings corroborate research literature on racial identity levels (Helms & Piper, 1994) that state that even during the process whereby White racist identities are abandoned (contact-reintegration), an individual may harbor pro-White attitudes, view Blacks in stereotypically negative terms, and feel fearful, angry, and hostile toward Blacks (reintegration phase).

In contraposition to the empathic failures of an anticlient perspective, the proclient position may draw heavily on principles associated with working within the Real Relationship, in this regard adopting a phenomenological, nonjudgmental and humanistic perspective. Participants operating from a proclient perspective recognized that when clients were from contexts unfamiliar to their own, effective therapy might be facilitated if a safe, containing space were provided for the exploration of client affect and if client meaning systems were empathically tracked. While overemphasis of the humanistic perspective can detract from social realities (Cloete & Pillay, 1988; Turton 1986), a humanistic focus may also encourage therapists exposed to apartheid ideology to raise racial issues directly while disregarding negative racial stereotypes. In short, the proclient position encourages counselors to connect on a personal level rather than responding to a racial label.

A common theme in the interview data was the importance of positive regard, warmth, and genuineness, coupled with effective interpretation and confrontation of clients. As noted by Pedersen (1977, 1978, 2000) in his development of the Triad Model, taking care to establish a correct balance between client-accommodative positive regard, on the one hand, and more confrontative techniques on the other, may help to establish a Working Alliance and promote healing when working with clients from different social groups.

The empathic failure and therapy-hindering consequences of the anticlient position stand in opposition to the proclient promotion of such therapeutic relationships as the Working Alliance or the Real Relationship. Self-awareness, intimacy, emotional joining, nondefensiveness and a nonpejorative approach were dominant values that therapists believed were facilitating of effective interracial therapy.

Another relationship type that therapists stated they might use to facilitate interracial therapy was the Transferential/Countertransferential Relationship. Some of the therapists, influenced by psychodynamic conceptualizations, stated that they invited the transference and explored how the client experienced the therapist as a White person, in order to explicate interracial dynamics and assist in the unlearning of stereotypes. These psychodynamically oriented therapists also stated a need to be aware of their own countertransferences. The study substantiated an important role in interracial therapy for countertransference feelings that literature has suggested could:

1. inform a therapist about how other people perceive and relate to the client; and
2. inform therapists of their own prejudices
    (Moosa, 1992; Peebles-Kleiger, 1989; Racker, 1957; Sandler et al., 1970).

Whether therapists choose to work in the Transferential/Countertransferential Relationship, the Real Relationship, the Working Alliance or any other relationship modality is often a matter of paradigmatic allegiance as well as an evaluation of clinical appropriateness. An important contribution of the study was its differentiation between healing relationships in general and therapy-hindering practices. While the anticlient position creates barriers between therapists and clients, the proclient position aims to promote healing through the establishment of a strong therapy relationship, no matter the therapist's paradigmatic allegiances.

Subordination Versus the Advancement of Dignity

Whitecentric perspectives lead to a position where Blacks are viewed as different, inferior, and subordinate in therapy. The anticlient position is characterized by excesses or abuses of power such as minimizing clients' autonomy by excluding them from decision-making processes, and using stigmatizing, deficit-oriented labels. The training and practice of counselors that frequently fails to accommodate other beliefs can result in client oppression (Hickson, Christie, & Shmukler, 1990). The study substantiated observations that White counselors may lose sight of Black clients as individuals when they automatically ascribe problems to difficulties of cultural and racial conflict (Vontress, 1971, p. 9). Therapists' conscious or unconscious beliefs in White supremacy and a belief that the patient's problems are an outgrowth of his or her inferiority may, as noted by Greene (1985, p. 392), lead to paternalistic, patronizing behavior. Participants in the study referred to potentially subordinating factors such as "a total power imbalance" between White therapists who take on the role of the authority figure and Black clients who are in a subordinate position. In these instances, relations of domination were seen as almost inevitable as epitomized in doctor expert versus patient deferring roles.

White psychologists comprise a particularly powerful elite. The White group has been historically advantaged, has had the power to control other groups, and has exercised that power. Moreover, the knowledge possessed by psychologists represents a considerable source of power that is amplified by their legally and socially mandated interventions in matters pertaining to mental health. When exercised from an anticlient base, the power of mental health practitioners can lead to client dependency on therapist dictates and the subservience of Black clients to subordinating White practices. The proclient position, on the other hand, facilitates the advancement of dignity and autonomy for all clients. Influenced by an ideology of racial sensitivity and the influence of human rights perspectives, the proclient position advances appeals for personal and group rights, empowerment, nonsubjugation and client respect.

Anxiety, Guilt, and Fear Versus Realistic Hope and Confidence

In addition to the dichotomy between anticlient Whitecentricism and proclient adherence to equality in diversity, a further categorization can be made between proclient hope and anticlient anxiety, guilt and fear. Realistic hope means that counselors believe in the potential benefits of interracial therapy without either minimizing its difficulties or overexaggerating the benefits of therapy. Belief that one is able to make a difference typifies the proclient position. Therapists operating from a proclient position expressed faith in their abilities to be of assistance to Black clients and, while recognizing that there may be difficulties in interracial therapy, avoided overfocusing on contextual difficulties to the point of becoming debilitated by anxiety. Their positive outlook, tempered with a healthy dose of realism, was one of the most significant factors differentiating the proclient position from negative anticlient feelings.

From an anticlient perspective, counselors' uncertainty as to the applicability and effectiveness of psychological theory and practice in African contexts may erode their confidence and lead to anxiety in interracial settings. In many instances, the study participants' exposure to apartheid ideology and racial segregation led to feelings of anxiety in interracial contexts. Contact in social situations that enhance awareness of group identification and fortify boundaries between groups may strengthen group identity fixation (Bornman & Appelgryn, 1999). The findings substantiated that a lack of social contact with Blacks on an equal footing undermines therapists' confidence to interact freely in interracial contexts.

The study further revealed that some White counselors might fear discreditation through Black clients perceiving them as unaware of the life circumstances of Black people and as ignorant of Black social milieus. The following interview extract provides an example of this concern:

I think they perceive me as possibly being elitist, as being the product of an advantaged product of the apartheid era. I perhaps feel that they come into the therapy thinking that she doesn't know enough about us culturally, that she doesn't understand, that she's not Black and, therefore, how does she know what it is like to be Black and to experience life as a Black and how that impacts emotionally on one's well-being?

Counselor anxiety that clients and therapists come from different cultural backgrounds, and that culture defines the person, were sometimes accompanied by concerns that cultural differences are not manageable and that differences between therapists and clients cannot be surpassed. Moreover, some of the counselors stated that they felt overwhelmed when dealing with issues of Black hardship. Their self-doubt was informed by concern as to whether they were able to fully comprehend the degree of adversity and the type of traumas that have been experienced by many Black South Africans.

Appropriate Challenge Versus Overcompensation

The anxiety of White therapists has a number of potentially negative consequences for effective interracial therapy. Concerns that they will be unable to establish rapport with Black clients may lead some therapists to become inhibited and unspontaneous; for other therapists their anxiety may lead to excessive talking that dominates psychotherapy sessions and deprives clients of working space.

Another aspect to White anxiety which emerged from the interviews is that White therapists may desist from confronting their clients even when it is therapeutically appropriate to do so, either because they feel sorry for them or because they want to avoid conflict with a member of another racial group. White therapists who feel guilty about their membership of a privileged and dominating group may overcompensate in interracial therapy by not challenging their Black clients where they would normally challenge a White client. Their painstakingly, nonjudgmental, placatory and sympathetic approach toward clients may disempower clients from mobilizing inner resources and inhibit spontaneity in a session.

Excessive guilt may inhibit the courage that is required to envisage and pursue valued goals (Erikson, 1963, 1964). In interracial contexts, psychotherapy could be restricted by counselors' countertransferential feelings of guilt. Three types of countertransferential guilt identified by Moosa (1992) in her study of trauma-workers' reactions in an overtly political context could also characterize the Anticlient position; viz:

1.   racial guilt;
2.   guilt associated with the privileges of class and race; and
3.   guilt at being relatively cocooned from the trials and tribulations suffered by patients.

In Moosa's study, several therapists appeared to consider their patients' trust as unearned or undeserved. In the Proclient-Anticlient study (Strous & Eagle, in process), an element of self-pity underpinned the therapists' concerns that they would be negatively perceived by Black clients or that they were confronted by overwhelming issues of negative life circumstances. Guardedness and inhibited spontaneity on the part of some White therapists were revealed to be based on concerns that their Black clients would perceive them negatively. As stated by two of the participants, under certain circumstances: "awareness ... of how damaged Black-White relationships have been in this country and still are ... could ... become a hindrance...it can be detrimental to the therapy to always just try keep things pleasant and nice." "Being too accommodating ... could stop the process of the therapy, of what we are really there to do."

Counselors' fears of realistic confrontation or oversympathetic treatment of clients who have suffered racial and social injustices may hinder therapy by detracting from a need for client change. In South Africa, where apartheid has come to be viewed as clearly inhumane and reprehensible, counselors may also feel that Black anger is legitimate; and in this sense, they may avoid triggering an expression of affect against which they do not feel they can defend themselves. There is a further possibility, as noted by Greene (1985), that therapists' fears that their own racism may leak out into treatment can result in a failure or reluctance to set appropriate limits or to interpret client acting-out.

Whereas overcompensation has deleterious, anticlient consequences, counselors operating from a proclient perspective of confidence are able to appropriately challenge clients, no matter their race. One of the participants, for instance, provided an example of how he had confronted his client's subservience as a Black woman in her therapy. Confronting contradictions, discrepancies or inconsistencies, exposing clients' secondary gains, reframing clients' defensiveness as countertherapeutic forms of control, and confronting resistance are important therapy-facilitating skills, especially in interracial contexts (Ridley, 1995).

Motivation Versus Disinvestment

Counselors are frequently involved in counseling people on intensely upsetting issues that place demands upon their own emotional resources. A strong theme that emerged was that a lack of external backup because of funding cuts or poor infrastructure contributed to therapists feeling unsupported and personally depleted.

The extent of poverty in the South African Black community at large and a shortage of resources and funds for mental health services exacerbated counselors' feelings of being overwhelmed. In order to protect themselves from these feelings, as well as from uncomfortable feelings of anxiety, guilt, or fear, several of the counselors indicated that they have tended to distance themselves from interracial contexts and Black clients. Feelings of helplessness and disillusionment in the face of seemingly overwhelming difficulties have frequently resulted in anticlient disinvestment and detachment. For example, one participant stated that in the absence of adequate infrastructural support she had experienced burn-out and "couldn't do it anymore;" she experienced a need to take time out from working with low-socio-economic class clients and restricted herself to working with clients who could afford private practice rates. As noted by Gibson, Sandenbergh, and Swartz (2001), psychologists may become disillusioned or feel that they do not possess the necessary skills or understanding to engage effectively in complex situations of a frightening and unfamiliar terrain. Psychologists are often exposed to violence in community settings, the effects of which are exacerbated by a lack of familiar cues on which to base their assessment of risk, possible language difficulties and difficulty accessing help from community members, and fantasy fears related to entering township areas, which apartheid presented as being off limits to them (Gibson, Sandenbergh, and Swartz, 2001).

In contradiction to anticlient disinvestment, a proclient approach results in therapist motivation in interracial contexts. Interracial therapy is facilitated when counselors do not experience debilitating anxiety, guilt, and fear or when they manage to overcome their debilitating effects. It is possible for counselors to glean important information from even their negative initial reactions to clients and /or situations, and they can put this information to good use. For instance, counselors' feelings of anger toward a group of patients could be considered a form of concordant countertransference—a direct experience of the sense of injustice and outrage to which their clients may have been subjected—with positive implications for counselor empathy when counselors are aware of their significance (Moosa 1992). There were many expressions of counselor outrage at injustices perpetrated against Blacks. These feelings could facilitate enhanced understanding and empathy on the part of counselors if they were appropriately attended to. One participant, for instance, stated that her abhorrence for the arrogance of Whites who facilitated cultural and racial oppression had helped sensitize her to the need for flexibility and to accept others' norms when engaging in interracial therapy.

If, as contended by Ridley (1995), racism is behavior that can be voluntarily controlled, and it is the responsibility of every mental health professional to combat racism, a proclient commitment to interracial therapy represents a moral victory over anticlient disinvestment and withdrawal. Effective counselors do not succumb to feelings of disillusionment. They have faith in interracial counseling and are motivated to try overcoming difficulties.

Ambivalence and Negotiation

The Anticlient-Proclient Model of Therapist Ambivalence (Figure 3) divides the anticlient position into two classifications:

1. Whitecentricism, and
2. Counselor anxiety, guilt and fear.

As seen, Whitecentricism results in processes of exclusion from full participation in the mental health care system, professional elitism, inflexibility, empathic failure, and client subordination. Anxiety, guilt, and fear lead to processes of overcompensation and disinvestment.

The proclient position has also been divided into two classifications, which stand in counter-position to the anticlient position:

1. Equality in diversity, and
2. Realistic hope and confidence.

Belief in equality in diversity results in processes that promote healing and dignity and that are inclusive, consultative, and flexible. Realistic hope and confidence result in processes of appropriate client challenge, and counselor motivation to engage in interracial therapy.

Although there are sustained and compelling themes that can be categorized into anticlient and proclient positions, a common trend is for interviewees to move backward and forward between different perspectives. A sustained analysis of the interviews revealed processes of vacillation and shifting perspectives in the participants' accounts. Ambivalence informed by competing ideological inputs and also based on debate concerning what strategies are best for clients, resulted in constant adjustments by therapists as they balanced up the pros and cons of seemingly contradictory perspectives. The negotiation of anticlient and proclient sentiments was frequently a fluid and iterative process, as counselors fluctuated in their allegiances to different ideological influences and as they tried to reconcile theoretical and practical dilemmas.

A factor contributing to shifts in the nature of their talk may have been counselor defensiveness and discursive rhetoric that concealed their true feelings. Nevertheless, reluctance to reveal true feelings is not a sufficient explanation. Notwithstanding the masking of anticlient sentiment, there was significant evidence of therapists sincerely trying to achieve a balance between seemingly contradictory perspectives. Counselors' shifting and contradictory perspectives during the interviews reflected processes of self-questioning or conscientizing that occurred in the process of the interview dialogue.

There were suggestions in the interviews that overemphasis of proclient or anticlient sentiment by a therapist may result in that therapist re-evaluating his or her position and entertaining the opposite position. One participant for instance, described how too much proclient sentiment could lead to anticlient positions. In her case, a pollyanyish approach, which did not acknowledge reality-based difficulties in interracial therapy, lead to unrealistic expectations and eventual burnout and disillusionment. Sentiment that might normally be regarded as proclient (faith in interracial therapy) can lead to anticlient sentiment when it is overexaggerated.

The exaggeration of anticlient sentiment may, vice versa, lead to proclient articulations. An interesting aspect of counselors' shifting perspectives was that *in vivo* exposure to Black clients during therapy might result in a reduction of anticlient sentiment and an increase in proclient sentiment as therapy progresses.

Social situations provide a multiplicity of perspectives that are continually negotiated and renegotiated (Gergen & Gergen, 1988; Mkhize & Frizelle, 2000) and counselors weighing up the relative pros and cons of competing anticlient and proclient positions fluctuate and flip-flop in a dialectical process. Apart from their exposure to different ideological influences that could be considered anticlient or proclient, particularly racist ideologies and competing democratic principles, counselors were faced with the following additional dilemmas.

A sameness-difference dilemma frequently confused therapists. In this regard, the interviewees frequently entertained competing visions of a universalist-particularist debate in relation to whether to assign importance to racial issues or whether to treat Black and White clients the same. For instance, a frequently stated quandary was whether one should challenge Black clients less than White clients in order to compensate for the Black experience of oppression by Whites. These dilemmas mirror similar debates in the literature (e.g., Draguns, 1989; Kottler, 1990). The etic approach is characterized by the adoption of a universalist perspective that emotional needs are constant across (and minimally influenced by) cultural, ethnic, or racial reference groups; with the implication that therapy as practiced in the West is universally applicable. In contrast, the fundamental assumption of an emic approach is that norms and expectations vary across cultures and social contexts and that different therapeutic frameworks are required in different contexts. In practice, the notion of a culture-free (universal) etic has been just as elusive as a culture pure emic (Pedersen, 2000a, p. 36). A perspective that combines the general and the specific viewpoints is required (Pedersen, 2000a, p. 37), but the study points to the often difficult process of balancing contradictory perspectives and counselors' concerns as to where to draw the lines between universalist and particularist contexts.

A related dilemma, reflected in both the interviews and the literature, centers on the appropriateness of middle class therapies with clients from lower socio-economic classes (e.g., Dawes, 1986; Hayes, 1986, Turton, 1986). In countries such as South

Africa, where racism resulted in widespread deprivation of opportunities for Blacks, issues of race and class have coincided with processes of oppression. In the interviews, many of the participants used the terms race, culture, and class interchangeably. Notwithstanding rhetorical processes that mask racism, and, which will be discussed shortly, the terminology used suggests that for many therapists race is an insufficient descriptor of demographic attributes in interracial therapy. More significantly, the appropriateness of interventions reflecting class encapsulation needs to be considered in interracial therapy because institutionalized racism frequently results in economic disadvantage.

Which counseling approaches are best suited for working class clients is a polemic. Long-term psychotherapy, such as psychodynamic interventions, have been criticized as ignoring the need for practical skills because of their focus on intrapsychic conflict (Ridley, 1995). Ridley (p. 47) contends that long-term psychotherapy is a largely unaffordable endeavor that is in any event watered down when applied to disempowered group members. Behavior therapy, which aims at practical behavioral change, has been accused of allowing therapists too much power and control, turning working-class clients into objects of manipulation. Client-centered approaches may permit greater client autonomy, rapport building, and emotional joining because of their nonjudgmental, phenomenological underpinnings, but they neglect social concerns (Cloete & Pillay, 1986).

Controversy surrounding the appropriateness of the various therapies to working class contexts is compounded by individual therapists' allegiances to different paradigmatic frames. Different schools of psychology adhere to diverse ontological and epistemological positions and frequently understand the requirements of working class clients differently. Moreover, South Africa is increasingly becoming a society in which class is no longer uniform amongst all Black people or among all White people. Recognition of clients' varying class levels could represent a differentiated appreciation of race and has implications for how interracial therapy is conducted.

Another debate that confronted therapists was between structuralist accounts that view personality as intact and difficult to change, and poststructuralist accounts that emphasize ongoing change. Structuralist leanings underscored a number of the anticlient themes. For instance, the view of Blacks as likely to be both the victims and perpetrators of aggression because of experiences of community violence, and the view of a national level narcissistic injury leading to feelings of entitlement, carried implications of personality traits that are difficult to treat. In contradiction to such deficit-oriented formulations, poststructuralist approaches reject the legitimacy of deterministic evaluations that deny the continual cocreation of Self (L. Richardson, 1994).

As a further example of the structuralist-poststructuralist debate, a quandary alluded to by several of the participants was the extent to which Black clients and family structures have been adversely affected by oppression and disrupted family life. Some participants mentioned that a psychodynamic focus on the nuclear family raised difficulties when formulating clinical impressions. In particular, a perspective of African children as deprived and families as broken because working class parents were absent, having left home to work, could be inaccurate because of the availability of alternative adequate caregivers such as grandparents. An appreciation of alternative lifestyles rejects dominant value judgments and hegemonic knowledge, but it may be shortsighted for therapists to ignore social processes that have in many in-stances undermined family life.

In summary, both the study and the literature point to a number of dilemmas fac-ing counselors in interracial contexts. The appropriateness of bourgeois counseling, universalist-particularist dilemmas, structuralist-poststructuralist debates and the competing demands of anticlient and proclient perspectives require counselors to entertain and frequently adjust to contradictory and competing perspectives. Shifting attitudes towards these and related dilemmas reflect that therapists' talk tends to fluc-tuate during the negotiation of contradictory perspectives. Our discussion now turns to how this dialogical flip-flop process can be harnessed with positive benefits for improved counselor insight and reduced resistance to acknowledging the potential for subtle racism.

Improved Insight

It was anticipated that counselors asked to evaluate an exercise requiring them to grapple with the likely resolutions of their therapy-facilitating proclient talk and their therapy-hindering anticlient talk would express a heightened sensitivity to and a more sophisticated understanding of the influence of racial attitudes in interracial counseling contexts. Following the interviews, in which their therapy-hindering and therapy-facilitating attitudes were gleaned via open-ended questions as well as through personified anticlient and proclient role-plays, a number of the participants reported that they had found the exercise thought provoking and growth producing. Some of the responses received from the participating psychologists were, in indi-vidual cases, that the role-plays increased their awareness of:

1. their own racist tendencies;
2. their propensity to overcompensate for feelings of anxiety, fear, and guilt by not chal-lenging Black clients where they would challenge White clients;
3. their tendency to intellectualize about interracial therapy without actually engaging in it,
4. their propensity to disinvest from interracial counseling because of their own feelings of discomfort;
5. personal allegiances to racial sensitivity and feelings of empathy which facilitate in-terracial therapy and which contradict anticlient elements, and;
6. a desire to engage more in interracial therapy contexts.

The participants' increased awareness following the interviews constituted an ad-vance over ideological closure, which limits choice (Habermas, 1990b; Ingleby, 1981; Painter & Theron, 1998). Insight, as a form of awareness, permits one to grasp the unity of disparate elements in a field. The person who is aware knows *what* he or she does, *how* he or she does it, that there are alternatives, and that he or she *chooses* to be a certain way (Simkin & Yontef, 1984, p. 290). Moreover, "awareness is ac-companied by *owning*, that is, the process of knowing one's control over, choice over, responsibility for, one's own behavior and feelings" (Simkin & Yontef, 1984).

The participating counselors' increased self-awareness and insight suggest a beneficial role for a model that juxtaposed their therapy-hindering and therapy-facilitating attitudes and practices in order to permit access to disparate facets of in-ner dialogue in interracial contexts. As a result of the interviews and the personified role plays, which required them to negotiate competing anticlient and proclient sen-

timents, most of the participants reported a heightened sensitivity to, and a more sophisticated understanding of, the effects of racial attitudes in interracial contexts.
Entering into dialogue with a multiplicity of voices or perspectives may lead to an
emergence of a clearer perspective of one's own (Hermans, 1996). It is gratifying
that a number of the counselors, as a result of insights gained during the interviews,
reported such sentiments as "wanting to try harder" with regard to interracial therapy.
As shall be discussed, the counselors' improved awareness of their personal ambivalences toward interracial therapy and their enhanced appreciation of the influence of
racial attitudes in interracial counseling contexts augurs well for improved counseling services.

Resistance to Exploring Anticlient Sentiment

Despite the overall evaluation of the interviews and role-plays as beneficial, some
of the participants found them stressful. These participants may have felt threatened
for the following reasons:

1. They may have been unwilling to access undesirable prejudices they hold on an un-
    conscious level;
2. They may have felt loathe and possibly ashamed to openly articulate politically incor-
    rect prejudices or racist tendencies;
3. They may have not wanted to reveal ignorance or lack of experience;
4. Their feelings of vulnerability may have escalated because of the anticlient role-
    plays, which forced self-analysis to a personal level beyond theoretical intellectuali-
    zation.

Therapist resistance against exploring issues of race and racism were evident in
such self-protective defense mechanisms as projection, intellectualization, denial,
and rationalization. These mechanisms warrant further scrutiny.

Projection

Counselor projection occurs in therapy when counselors unconsciously attribute
their own unacceptable impulses, attitudes, and behaviors to their clients. During the
interviews, there were a number of instances of counselors attributing their own undesirable attitudes toward interracial therapy to their Black clients. For instance, one
of the participant's concerns that her Black clients should be comfortable in interracial therapy reflected her own discomfort in interracial settings. As she conceded: "I
perhaps ignore ... diversity ... from the viewpoint of not trying to make the client
uncomfortable and yet ... I should in myself work towards containing the discomfort
and dealing with it better."

Fanon (1986a) has drawn on classical Freudian notions of projection to explain
the impulses of White racists to degrade, oppress, and dominate Blacks. Ethnic and
racial stereotypes provide a convenient target for the attribution of negative personal
characteristics (Adorno, Frenkel-Brunswick, Levinson, & Sanford, 1950). Projecting
negative personal characteristics onto others has the effect of scapegoating and alienating them, and provides a rationalization for their exclusion from the privileges reserved for dominant elites (Littlewood & Lipsedge, 1997; van Dijk, 1993).

Intellectualization

Despite emphasis being placed on the need for counselor self-awareness and emotional "working through," many therapists may be prone to intellectualization. Some of the participants pontificated about issues on a "head level" and conceded that they do not really experience them on an emotional or behavioral level. Intellectualizing about the need for racial inclusion, for instance, is a bland platitude if unaccompanied by commensurate action. One needs to walk the talk to be authentic.

The participants' paying of lip service to notions of multiculturalism is an example of talk that frequently occurred on an intellectual rather than a practical level. A difficulty with some appeals for multiculturalism is that talk about the need to be culturally sensitive may conceal a lack of factual engagement in nonracist practice. As a participating therapist suggested, discussing multiculturalism in intellectual terms could have been a cop-out for therapists who found it easier to discuss culture than race.

Another example of intellectualization in the interviews was the construction of pseudoscientific terminology to give credibility to points of view without attracting charges of racism. For example, intellectualizing about cultural differences might appear to be culturally sensitive while actually obscuring racial stereotyping and anticlient sentiment. Culture "is often confused with race both in common parlance and in professional thinking, mainly because people who are seen as racially different are conceptualized as having different cultures, and the term 'culture' is used to conceal racism" (Fernando, 1991, p. 22).

Denial

A denial defense may protect counselors from having to acknowledge ideological influences that have operated in the society in which they interact and that influence their anticlient sentiments. For instance, some of the interviewees found appeal in a color-blind position. Color-blindness in counseling—that is, the tendency to treat a client as if his or her color were of no consequence—permits silence on such issues as the unequal distribution of power in Black and White relations, and the racism that underpins anticlient counseling positions.

The participants frequently constructed therapy from a humanistic basis, as valuing human individuality and as being uncontaminated by racial issues. As much as humanistic perspectives avoid pejorative labeling, they tend to downplay social tensions. Therapists' "homogenization of racial differences" (Ridley, 1995) could be considered a form of social denial. During the interviews, many of the participants referred to their nonjudgmental stance, with the further implication that in therapy phenomenological tracking of Black clients can level social power imbalances. These references tended to overlook or remained silent on power inequalities and racial identity interactions, which frequently affect White counselor and Black client dyads (Helms, 1990, 1994).

Denial is a central element of racism in its newer guises (van Dijk, 1987). A frequent failure on the part of the counselors to mention relevant issues of social inequity was reflective of noncritical discourse that permits discursive reproductions of racism to continue unchallenged. Not allowing politically unpopular facts to be perceived, allowed into full awareness or acknowledged is a form of "social amnesia"

(Jacoby, 1975) or ideological denial that permits anticlient sentiment to remain covert.

Rationalization

Rationalization represents irrational behavior as rational in order to justify it to oneself and others. For instance, Whites who are frequently motivated to give a non-discriminatory self-presentation (Essed, 1991) may detract from important issues such as racism by providing reasons for its perpetuation. As an example of this, White counselors may exonerate themselves from treating Black patients in a more flexible and accommodative manner by rationalizing that the under-representation of Blacks in mental health services is understandable because these services are unsuitable or inappropriate to Afrocentric preferences and because traditional healers are available to minister to the mental health needs of Blacks. These arguments fail to insist on equal treatment options for Black clients and provide a rationalization for the exclusion of Blacks from therapy.

Rationalizations are "handy psychological tricks we use to get out of tight spots" (Hauck, 1990, p. 38). In the context of the study, seemingly plausible and acceptable reasons for therapists' conduct that could invite censure were often offered in conjunction with appeals for equal opportunity. As an example, affirmative action policies were repudiated with reference to the deleterious consequences of reverse discrimination against Whites, and failure to explore the worldview of Black clients was rationalized on the basis of a need to protect the counselor's own worldview. These rationalizations effectively supported the maintenance of White privilege, but within the context of advocating for human rights. The concept of affirmative action as necessary to address past injustices and to promote the quality and dignity of all South Africans has accumulated an enormous negative response in some sectors. A tendency to assume that affirmative action policies are only in the costs and not in the benefits of the scale fails to appreciate that affirmative action can play a powerful role in promoting legitimacy, efficiency, and growth (Albertyn and White, 1994). Symbolic racism includes antagonism towards mechanisms for redressing inequality (Seares, 1988). The articulation, by people who do not consider themselves racist, that blacks are becoming too demanding, that their needs are unfair, and that institutions are giving them more than they deserve is a form of modern racism (McConahay in Jones, 1997). White therapists who perceive that their way of doing things and its associated benefits are under threat may engage in conservative social practices and offer rationalizations weighted toward the maintenance of White privilege and away from Black empowerment.

Trivializing potential criticisms and discrediting their proponents is another way in which the participants sometimes defended their own privilege. This is in keeping with Essed's (1987) observations that White elites may depoliticize important social issues such as racism by referring to Blacks as too sensitive or that they may veil patronizing attitudes toward Blacks by trying to pacify them, claiming their good intentions, or expressing annoyance at Blacks' lack of gratitude for White benevolence (Essed, 1987). During the interviews, some of the participants who had expressed Whitecentric views further pathologized Black clients as likely perpetrators of rights violations, as "entitled," or as in some other way deficient. This form of victim blaming, in which racial victimization was attributed to the victims themselves, served to detract from the problem of Whitecentricism. For instance, some of the White counselors indicated that they took offence at suggestions that they could not appreciate the worldview of their clients. This is evident in the following extract: "I'm … angry because … the client wants me to provide something for nothing, which is part of the entitlement, at the same time as being contemptuous … in the sense that they assume that I can't understand where they're coming from, which makes me think "then what are you doing here?"

White elites frequently reject explicitly or blatantly racist ideologies, but fail to consider their own role in creating and defining the moderate mainstream (van Dijk, 1993). Counselors defend themselves against suggestions that they play a role in difficulties in interracial therapy through mechanisms such as rationalization, denial, intellectualization, and projection.

Therapists' Views of Themselves as Blameless for Therapy Difficulties

When counselors are defended against acknowledging their own potential for racism and/or encapsulation, it becomes extremely difficult to challenge anticlient positions without causing offence. Elites frequently define themselves as moral watchdogs, dissociate themselves from intentional racism, and defend themselves against any thesis that potentially disconfirms the normative self-concept of being nonracist (van Dijk, 1993). Consequently, conclusions of research on racism and accusations of disempowerment "are often denied, marginalized, or even violently attacked by the elites who thereby precisely confirm the plausibility of the thesis" (van Dijk, 1993, p. 9). One of the surest signs of racial defensiveness is when counselors try to convince themselves that they are not prejudiced (Ridley, 1995).

One of the most striking discursive features of the study interview transcripts was the sense that therapists, even if inadvertently, seem to hold clients primarily responsible for difficulties in interracial therapy—portraying themselves almost as hapless victims of clients' constructions or projections onto them. For example, several of the therapists implied that they could not help it if their clients cast them in the roles of "expert doctor," "White racist" or "beneficiary of apartheid." In addition to deficit understandings of Black clients linked to negative life circumstances and upbringing, these therapists' complaints constituted a form of blaming the other, and seemed to effectively place the burden of responsibility for both difficulties and solutions in interracial contexts on Black clients.

White therapists' portrayal of themselves as the victims of Black clients' unfair constructions and projections tends to fit with more covert manifestations of racism in which liberal sentiment argues that Whites who have been privileged nevertheless have rights that need protection. It is important to tackle but difficult to detect the subtle racism underlying constructions that are weighted more toward the maintenance of White's rights and less toward advocacy for Blacks' rights. Features of subtle racism, however, become more evident when anticlient and proclient dialogue is critically reflected upon.

Implications for Anticlient-Proclient Model Training

There are many examples of counselor talk, which, viewed from a hermeneutic of faith, appear to be culturally sensitive and benign, but, viewed from a hermeneutic of suspicion, reveal a more problematic side. White therapists may present themselves as having the best interests of Black patients at heart, and this may be the case in many instances. Their seeming and actual kindness may, however, obscure patronizing and intolerant attitudes and practices.

Therapists exposed to different ideological positions have ambivalent attitudes toward interracial therapy and tend to oscillate between anticlient and proclient positions. Emphasizing proclient perspectives may serve to detract attention from some of the anticlient perspectives held by therapists. Therefore, in order to arrive at a critical evaluation, therapists' self-talk should be interpreted from a hermeneutic of suspicion as well as phenomenologically. Otherwise, anticlient intolerance may be concealed behind a mask of proclient tolerance.

Covert anticlient sentiment reflects the insidious, ironic situation where White racism is "absent yet present" (Wong, 1994, p. 134). As Wong has stated: "'Whiteness' is about a topic within psychology that does not seem to exist but one whose power and presence are continuously felt. It is a subject that asserts its centrality or dominance on social and cultural levels yet remains shrouded within a veil of transparency that ensures its absence, thus evading the subject of discourse" (p. 136).

The Anticlient-Proclient Model provides a conceptually useful framework for the exploration of issues pertaining to White counselor identity. White elites, implicated in everyday racism through passivity, acquiescence, ignorance, and indifference, and through condoning or refraining from action against the discursive reproduction of racism (van Dijk, 1993), need to critically interrogate their own privileges and to break down prejudice and discrimination amongst themselves (Wong, 1994; Katz, 1982). Having as one of its goals a critically informed process of self-reflection, the Anticlient-Proclient Model is compatible with postmodernist and social constructionist appeals for researchers and therapists to closely scrutinize their feelings, biases, and personal peccadilloes (King, 1996).

Well-intentioned therapists may be unaware that they are behaving in racist ways because they have been socialized in racist societies in which the ideology of racism is largely unquestioned (Pedersen, 1997). The Anticlient-Proclient Model, which aims to articulate both the therapy-facilitating as well as the therapy-hindering self-talk of counselors in interracial counseling contexts, could play a positive role in increasing counselors' sensitivity to issues of race and racism and challenging taken-for-granted positions of ideological closure. The need to supplement the training of mental health professionals to take into account issues of race and racial identity may be well served by Anticlient-Proclient training.

The Anticlient-Proclient Model assumes that the personification of therapist attitudes in role-plays may lead to a more concretized awareness for therapists of their ambivalent attitudes toward interracial therapy. The analysis of the initial data supports this assumption and suggests that future development of the Anticlient-Proclient Model is warranted. Concretizing the antagonistic attitudes of therapists in interracial therapy, in the form of an anticlient personification, explicates therapist resistance as a real problem with ramifications beyond intellectual abstraction.

The initial results further suggest that the Anticlient-Proclient Model, which conceptualizes the anticlient position and the proclient position as standing in dialectical opposition to each other, could permit counselors in training to vacillate between different ideological perspectives. Flip-flopping between different positions holds open the possibility of increased appreciation for the dynamic relationships that exist between different levels of experience (Combrink-Graham, 1987). Following the argument of literary theorists such as Bakhtin (1981), when counselors enter into dialogue with a number of social and cultural voices they may be able to form their own voice based on a *selective* assimilation of the other voices. This would entail a process of "ideological becoming" (Bakhtin, 1981, p. 341). Authoritative discourse, which is monological, which refuses challenge, and which demands unconditional allegiance, may then be replaced by "internally persuasive discourse" (Bakhtin, p. 341), which emerges through processes of dialogical negotiation and renegotiation (Mkhize & Frizelle, 2000). There were many examples in the transcripts of counselors articulating points of view and then pausing to reflect on the validity of their articulations, apparently evidencing the kind of self-dialogue that Bakhtin refers to.

As with Pedersen's Triad Training Model, Anticlient-Proclient training may promote counselor growth without risk to actual clients. Simulated role-plays and group discussions following role-plays may provide counselors with immediate feedback as to the processual outcomes of competing anticlient and proclient positions. Group discussions may also serve to normalize for trainees that they are not alone in their entertainment of either anticlient or proclient sentiments. In fact, it is possible that group discussions will result in a piggyback process triggering the identification by therapists of anticlient and proclient sentiments of which they were consciously unaware.

Our thought processes belong to the core of ourselves and it is frequently difficult for people to admit that they may not be in control of them (Kohut, 1972, pp. 383-384). Therapists may therefore take offence and hurt at insinuations of racism, as was sometimes evident in the transcripts. While the anticlient role-plays resulted in anxiety for some of the counselors, a group training experience may help trainees to realize that they are not abnormal in their anticlient perspectives. For this to occur, it would be important to conduct group training in an atmosphere of nonjudgmental acceptance. Should a safe environment not be facilitated, it is highly probable that counselors' resistance to self-exploration and personal disclosure would be engaged.

Therapist resistance to articulating anticlient positions may be bypassed in Anticlient-Proclient training because the role-playing counselor does not have to directly articulate his or her own anticlient position. The anticlient literally puts words in the mouth of the counselor's personified therapy-hindering-part. Defensive counselors could save face by not articulating their own therapy-hindering attitudes personally, although later reflection may enable them to identify with the anticlient and to scrutinize their own anticlient positions.

The role-personification of anticlient sentiment could effect its linguistic separation from the personal identity of participating trainees. Perceptions of discontinuity between the role-played and the role-player may permit increased leakage of the self (Yardley, 1995) for later analysis when counselors are more ready to integrate emergent material.

The Anticlient-Proclient Model is based on an acknowledgment of the need to explicate the inner talk of people from different social groups when they interact with each other. It extends upon the Triad Model, which focuses on client self-talk, by providing for the articulation of counselor self-talk as well. The Anticlient-Proclient

Model therefore shifts the focus somewhat from *client* diversity to a greater emphasis on exploring *counselors'* attitudes. There are two benefits to this:

1. The Anticlient-Proclient design, unlike the Triad Model, requires no coached team apart from the trainees. This has advantages in terms of time, finances, and logistics. In more comprehensive training, the Anticlient-Proclient Model has the flexibility to incorporate coached persons should such incorporation be desired.
2. As was evident in the study, supposedly discrete groups have frequently been scrutinized based on assumptions concerning their apparent "otherness" (Swartz, 1987, p. 27). This is contradicted by training that places responsibility on counselors to explore their own prejudices. There is a need to move away from exotic perspectives in which certain groups are patronizingly treated as curiosities or inferior (Pedersen, 1988, 1991).

Both Triad Model training and Anticlient-Proclient training have benefits and may prove useful when sensitively applied. When combined, the two training techniques, incorporating anticounselor, anticlient, procounselor, and proclient combinations may facilitate awareness of client self-talk as well as counselors' own biases. In psychodynamic terms, the Triad Model may improve counselor insight into transference issues in intergroup contexts; the Anticlient-Proclient Model may increase insight into countertransference issues.

A particular advantage of the Anticlient-Proclient Model is that it does not focus on a one-sided criticism of counselor racism or inadequacy. An equal focus on the proclient position and its attendant underpinnings of counselor confidence and commitment to human rights provides a balance to the anticlient position. The identification of an ideology of human rights as confluent and concordant with effective interracial counseling could inspire a feeling in counselors that interracial therapy is a noble and worthwhile pursuit; and a trainer's empathic tracking of a trainee counselor's proclient perspectives may help to ameliorate that counselor's potential anxiety when anticlient perspectives are identified.

Anticlient-Proclient training may promote productive exploration of the threads linking ideological processes and the interventions of individual counselors. The Anticlient-Proclient Model's dual focus on counseling procedures that are either therapy-facilitating or therapy-hindering and the discussion of the historical and ideological antecedents of anticlient and proclient sentiments following role-plays may facilitate counselor's insight into the effects of socialization on their own counseling.

It therefore appears that the Anticlient-Proclient Model has potential to ameliorate and manage resistance to the exploration of therapy-hindering thoughts and feelings. The model also holds promise for the identification and exploration of therapy-facilitating thoughts and feelings. The interactive effects of these therapy-facilitating and therapy-hindering elements, observed and discussed in safe group workshops, could help counselors move toward greater awareness and more positive negotiation of their ambivalent attitudes toward interracial therapy. This would help to bridge the hiatus that exists between a need for counselors' self-insight when dealing with racially salient material and the limited training techniques that have been available to facilitate this, and could ultimately contribute to the delivery of more appropriate mental health services.

SUMMARY

The anticlient and proclient positions can be differentiated in terms of polarized characteristics. Counselors tend to weigh up the pros and cons of anticlient and proclient claims and to vacillate between these positions. Initial research suggests that the Anticlient-Proclient Model could prove useful in helping clients to track their ambivalent attitudes toward interracial therapy, to differentiate between their therapy-hindering and therapy-facilitating sentiments, and to understand the dialectic interplay between them.

Afterword

> The world in which the counselor went to school and had his (*sic*) early
> job experiences is no longer in existence. The more rapid the rate of
> change, the greater the gap between yesterday and tomorrow. It is most
> human indeed to "draw upon our experience" but of this the counselor
> must beware. Some of what we learnt may be for tomorrow but most of it
> remains for yesterday. (Wrenn, 1962, p. 448)

This cautionary warning, written as one of the first introductions to the notion of
counselor encapsulation, is as applicable today as it was when first written. Distorted
stereotypes of Black clients have always been inappropriate and are especially contradictory to democratic initiatives. However, the mental health professions have
frequently colluded in the mistreatment of disempowered groups, often because they
lack insight that they are doing so. Counselors may be unable to fully appreciate their
clients' worldviews because of their own ideologically constricted perspectives.

Interracial therapy involves complex dynamics. However, the inner thoughts and
feelings of psychotherapists or counselors pertaining to race are seldom articulated. It
is essential to the therapeutic endeavor for counselors to understand the impact of
their racially informed attitudes, the assumptions they make about their clients in
racial contexts, and how these potentially facilitate or interfere with therapeutic relationships.

In South Africa, therapists have been exposed to the competing values of apartheid ideology and racism, which denigrate Black people; psychological training,
which overtly teaches client respect (although the unbiased nature of psychology has
been challenged critically); and an increasingly popular focus on human rights.
These competing inputs result in ambivalent attitudes when dealing with racially
salient material. It is especially important in this country, which has been characterized by racial segregation and friction, to investigate attitudes of counselors when
dealing with racially salient material.

South African therapists who rely on schools of psychology imported from other
countries need to carefully ascertain the appropriateness of their practices, as well as
their personal biases that might have been influenced by apartheid structures. Already socialized within the milieu of a Whitecentered racist society, White South
African counselors have been inducted into a profession largely characterized by
decontextualised and desocialised notions of psychological theory and practice. In

South Africa, as elsewhere, insufficient exploration of racial identity has allowed mental health professionals to remain unaware of the therapeutic implications of an important social identity variable.

South Africa has gone through times of flux, from the dark days of apartheid oppression to having one of the most enlightened and democratic constitutions. Mirroring these processes of transformation, there has been and continues to be a need to substitute discriminatory mental health practices, previously accepted as conventional, with more culturally and racially sensitive alternatives. This has created opportunities to revisit the country's mental health system and counseling practices. In this book, apartheid-style psychology with its implications of exclusion, elitism, empathic failure, inflexibility, and oppression have been compared with perspectives conducive to racial and cultural tolerance. Many goals and practices of psychology are concordant with an ideology of human rights, and on a more positive note, counselors' attitudes of cultural and racial sensitivity compete with the disruptive, prejudicial attitudes, discriminatory practices, and truncated understandings that underpin apartheid-style psychology.

South Africa provides a special example of cultural intolerance on a widespread level. Institutionalized racism plagued South African society and found expression in the mental health field. Nevertheless, much of the literature referred to in this book is international. Worldwide, there is increasing recognition that human rights must be protected within mental health systems and counseling practices. Contextually unsuitable psychological strategies have often been used with members of nondominant groups, throughout the world. Mental health delivery for disempowered groups have often been wanting in comparison to facilities for White, middle-class, Eurocentric persons. Issues confronting South African counselors are in some ways unique, but they also resonate with international literature and experiences. Counselors should be considerate and compassionate with all people, and cultural and racial sensitivity in counseling is likely to grow as a global human rights issue.

Despite the need discussed in this book to explore counselors' attitudes in interracial counseling, there are limited techniques available for this. To worsen matters, issues of racial identity are frequently unconscious, or prove threatening to counselors' self-esteem when brought to their attention. In order to overcome this impasse, an extension to Paul Pedersen's Triad Model, in the form of an anticlient triad design and a proclient triad design, has been proposed. The Anticlient-Proclient Model, which explicates the self-talk of therapists in interracial and multicultural counseling contexts, warrants further research. Evaluations of antistereotyping workshops may be difficult to assess. Nevertheless, the development and execution of antiracist intervention programs such as the one proposed is important given the often covert nature of racism.

The elaboration of the Triad Model in the introduction of anticlient and proclient dialogue appears to offer a comprehensive training tool with potential to address many of the reflective needs of therapists in interracial counseling contexts. Modern forms of racism tend to be subtle, difficult to identify, and intractable. The proposed Anticlient-Proclient Model offers opportunities for therapists to challenge their own assumptions concerning interracial therapy, to shift responsibility away from deficit-oriented notions of client failure and to try stem the perpetuation of subtle racism in interracial counseling contexts. It is hoped that this will go some way towards contributing to the operationalization of a Human Rights agenda in the field of multicultural counseling.

For heuristic reasons, anticlient and proclient positions and their processual outcomes are presented as bipolar dimensions in this book. However, it is likely that counselors do not merely oscillate between discrete categories of anticlient and proclient dimensions. Counselors may integrate varying amounts of anticlient and proclient sentiment at different stages. The investigation of the degrees of anticlient and proclient sentiment that may dominate counselors' racial identity levels may be suited to quantitative analyses of numerical data.

It needs to be acknowledged that notions of race and racism are not static. They tend to change over time and in different contexts. Moreover, "each generation can only go so far before it is stymied by its own psychological limitations" (Richards, 1998, p. 181). Future evaluations of counselors' self-talk in interracial contexts will therefore be necessary, and will hopefully contribute accounts that improve upon the present one.

The potential advantages and/or disadvantages of conducting Anticlient-Proclient training in mixed racial groups are unclear and warrant consideration. An interesting possibility would be to have the roles of counselor, anticlient and proclient played by members of different racial groups. Another possibility would be to hold debriefing sessions in which members of different racial groups cooperate in reflecting on their observations of the role-plays.

As important as it is to deal with issues of Whitecentricism, an obvious limitation has been the present focus on White counselors and Black clients. Black counselor and White client interactions may also benefit from conceptual analyses based on anticlient and proclient understandings. Interactions between members of other racial groups could also be investigated.

Another limitation of this book is its reliance on terms of racial classification. Race is a social construct. To ignore the visibility of race and the traditional assignment of people to, or their identification with, different racial groups, would be to ignore the historical and factual realities of their experiences. The term "race" has important interpersonal and intrapersonal implications and has been used here in a critically reflective sense to make Whiteness detectable and to unpack its problematic features, rather than to give credence to the dominator. The book, nevertheless, replicates a common occurrence in the literature in that it criticizes the concept of race on the one hand, and relies on it on the other. Perhaps only once issues of discrimination and privilege based on race cease to operate, will such dilemmas of terminology cease.

In the endeavor for improved counselor awareness, the need for accelerated inclusion of Blacks in the mental health care system, both as clients and as practitioners, must not be lost sight of. The training of therapists for improved racial awareness is important, but awareness alone is not sufficient. Commitment to a more equitable distibution of power and equal opportunity structures in mental health needs to be our ultimate goal.

Significant pointers have emerged that suggest that the Anticlient-Proclient Model could be beneficial in the training of counselors for improved racial sensitivity. It is therefore left to recommend that the model's possibilities should be explored. The development of training procedures for racial and cultural sensitivity training is an imperative, as evidenced by the types of issues that have emerged from the discussion of apartheid-style psychology and its more favorable alternatives.

References

Abas, M., Broadhead, J., Blue, I., Lewis, G. & Araya, R. (1995) Health service and community based responses to mental ill health in urban areas. In T. Harpham & I. Blue (eds.), *Urbanization and Mental Health in Developing Countries* (pp. 227-248). Aldershot: Avenburg.

Abdi, V.O. (1975). The problems and prospects of psychology in Africa. *International Journal of Psychology, 10*(3), 227-234.

Adams, M. (1997). Individualism, moral autonomy, and the language of human rights. *South African Journal on Human Rights, 13*(4), 501-513.

Adams, P.L. (1970). Dealing with racism in biracial psychiatry. *Journal of the American Academy of Child Psychiatry, 9,* 33-43.

Adams, W.A. (1950). The Negro patient in psychiatric treatment. *American Journal of Orthopsychiatry, 20,* 305-310.

Adorno, I., Frenkel-Brunswick, E., Levinson, D., & Sanford, R. (1950). *The Authoritarian Personality.* New York: Harper & Row.

Ahia, C.E. (1984). Cross cultural counseling concerns. *Personnel and Guidance Journal, 62,* 339-341.

Akin-Ogundeji,O. (1991). Asserting psychology in Africa. *The Psychologist: Bulletin of the British Psychological Society, 4,* 2-4.

Albertyn, C. & White, W. (1994). Germinating gender issues: Gender and affirmative action. *People Dynamics,* September 1994, 57-63.

Allen, B. (1971). Implications of social reaction research for racism. *Psychological Reports, 29,* 883-891.

American Association for the Advancement of Science (AAAS). (1990). *Mission of Inquiry Apartheid Medicine,* 52.

American Psychological Association (1992). Ethical principles of psychologists and code of conduct. *American Psychologist, 47,* 1612-1628.

American Psychiatric Association (1994). *Diagnostic and Statistical Manual of Mental Disorders* (4th ed.). Washington D.C.: APA.

American Psychiatric Association (APA). Committee on South Africa (1979*). American Journal of Psychiatry,* 136.

Anastasi, A. (1976*). Psychological Testing* (4th ed.). NY: Macmillan.

Andersen, S. M. & Miranda, R. M. (2000). Transference: How past relationships emerge in the present. *The Psychologist, 13, (*12), 608-609.

Anonymous (1986). Some thoughts on a more relevant or indigenous counseling psychology in South Africa: Discovering the socio-political context of the oppressed. *Psychology in Society, 5*, 81-89.

Appelbaum, K. (1998). Unpublished lecture to the postgraduate training course, Integrative Psychotherapy Association (South Africa), at the University of the Witwatersrand, Johannesburg.

Arrigo, B.A. & Williams, C.R. (1999). Chaos theory and the social control thesis—a post-Foucauldian analysis of mental illness and involuntary civil confinement. *Social Justice, 26*(1), 177-207.

Ashmore, R.D (1970). Solving the problem of prejudice. In B.E. Collins (ed.) *Social Psychology: Social Influence, Attitude Change, Group Processes, and Prejudice* (pp. 297-339). Reading, MA: Addison-Wesley.

Assagioli, R. (1965) *Psychosynthesis: A Manual of Principles and Techniques*. London: Aquarian/Thorsons.

Atkinson, D.R.; Morten, G. & Sue, D.W. (eds.), (1993). *Counseling American Minorities: A Cross-Cultural Perspective* (4th ed.). Madison, WI: W.L. Brown & Benchmark.

Auerbach, F. (1965). *The Power of Prejudice in South African Education*. Cape Town: Balkema.

Augustinos, M. & Walker, I. (1995). *Social Cognition: An Integrated Introduction*. London: Sage.

Avineri, S., & De-Shalit, A. (1992). Introduction. In S. Avineri & A. De-Shalit (eds.), *Communitarianism and Individualism* (pp. 1-11). New York: Oxford University Press.

Axelson, J.A. (1985). *Counseling and Development in a Multi-Cultural Society*. Monterey, CA: Brooks/Cole.

Bakker, T (1996). A postmodern mouse in the house of family therapy: The Eighth World Congress of the International Family Therapy Association. *Family Therapy Review* (ed. Shuda and Mason). South African Institute of Marital and Family Therapy.

Bailey, F.M. (1981). Cross-cultural counselor education: The impact of microcounseling paradigms and traditional classroom methods on counselor trainee effectiveness. Ph.D. Dissertation. University of Hawaii.

Bakhtin, M.M. (1973). *Problems of Doestevsky's Poetics* (2nd ed.) (Transl. R.W. Rotsel). Ann Arbor, MI: Ardis (originally published 1929).

Bakhtin, M.M. (1981). *The Dialogic Imagination* (C. Emerson & M. Holquist, trans.). Austin: University of Texas Press.

Barnes, E.J. (1980). The black community as the source of positive self-concept for black children: A theoretical perspective, In R.L. Jones (ed.), *Black Psychology* (2nd ed.). New York: Harper and Row.

Barry, T. & Guilfoyle, M. (1998). Second order cybernetics as a model for supervision. In L. Schlebusch (ed.), *South Africa Beyond Transition: Psychological Well-Being*. Proceedings of the 3rd Annual Congress of the Psychological Society of South Africa. (pp. 7-9). Pretoria: PsySSA.

Bassa, F M & Schlebusch, L (1984). Practice preferences of clinical psychologists in South Africa. *South African Journal of Psychology*.

Bateson, G. (1944). Cultural determinants of personality. In J. Hunt (ed.), *Personality and the Behavior Disorder* (pp. 723-730). New York: Roneod Press.

Beck, A. (1976). *Cognitive Therapy and Emotional Disorders*. New York: International Universities Press.

Beck, J. (1973). *The Counselor and Black/White Relations*. Boston: Houghton-Mifflin.

Bender, M.P. (1976). *Community Psychology*. Great Britain: Mathuen.

Bennett, L. (1966). *Before the Mayflower: History of the Negro in America, 1619-1964*. New York: Macmillan.

Berger, S. & Lazarus, S. (1987). The views of community organizers on the relevance of psychological practice in South Africa. *Psychology in Society, 7*, 6-23.

Bernstein, R.J. (1983). *Beyond Objectivism and Relativism: Science, Hermeneutics, and Praxis*. Philadelphia: University of Pennsylvania Press.

Berk, L.E. (1994). Why children talk to themselves. *Scientific American, 271*(6): 60-65.

Berne, E. (1961). *Transactional Analysis in Psychotherapy*. New York: Grove Press.

Bevis, W.M. (1921). Psychological traits of the Southern Negro with observations as to some of his psychoses. *American Journal of Psychiatry, 1*, 69-78.

Bidol, P. (1971). *Reflections of Whiteness in a White Racist Society* (pamphlet). Detroit: PACT.

Biesheuvel, S. (1987). Psychology, science, and politics: Theoretical developments and applications in a plural society. *South African Journal of Psychology, 17*, 1-8.

Billington,T.(1995). Discourse analysis: Acknowledging interpretation in everyday practice. *Education Psychology in Practice*, 11, 36-45.

Bion, W.R. (1957). Differentiation of the psychotic from the nonpsychotic personalities. *International Journal of Pscho-Analysis, 38*, 266-275.

Bion, W.R. (1962). *Learning from Experience*. London: Heinemann.

Bloom, L. (1994). Ethnic identity: A psychoanalytic critique. *Psychology in Society, 19*, 18-30.

Bloombaum, M, Yamamoto, J & James, A. (1968). Culture stereotyping among psychotherapists. *Journal of Consulting and Clinical Psychology 32*, 99.

Bodibe, R.C. (1993). What is the truth? Being more than just a jesting Pilate in South African psychology. *South African Journal of Psychology, 23* (2), 53-58.

Bodibe, R.C & Sodi, T. (1997). Indigenous healing. In Foster, D., Freeman, M., & Pillay, Y. (eds.). *Mental Health Policy Issues for South Africa*. Medical Association of South Africa.

Boonzaier, E. & Sharp, J. (eds). (1998). *South African Keyword: The Use and Abuse of Political Concepts*. Cape Town: David Philip.

Bornman, E. & Appelgryn, A. (1999). Predictors of ethnic identification in a transitory South Africa. *South African Journal of Psychology, 29* (2), 53-61.

Boscolo, Z.L., Cecchin, G., Campbell, D., & Draper, R. (1985). Twenty more questions—selections from a discussion between the Milan Associates and editors. In Campbell, D. and Draper, R. (eds.), *Applications of Systemic Family Therapy: The Milan Approach*. London: Grune & Stratton.

Bourdieu, P. & Passeron, J. (1977) *Reproduction in Education, Society and Culture*. London: Sage.

Boyer, L. (1989). Countertransference and techniques in working with the regressed patient: Further remarks. *International Journal of Psychoanalysis, 70*, 701-714.

Boynton, G. (1987). Cross-cultural family therapy: The escape model. *The American Journal of Family Therapy, 15*(2), 123-130.

Brabender, V. (1987). Vicissitudes of countertransference in inpatient psychotherapy. *International Journal of Group Psychotherapy, 37*, 549-567.

Bracero, W. (1994). Developing culturally sensitive psychodynamic case formulations: The effects of Asian cultural elements on psychoanalytic control-mastery theory. *Psychotherapy, 31*, 525-532.

Brislin, R.W. (1981). *Cross-Cultural Encounters*. New York: Pergamon.

Bruner, J. (1986). *Actual Minds, Possible Worlds*. Cambridge, MA: Harvard University Press.

Bryson, S. & Bardo, H. (1975). Race and counseling process: An overview. *Journal of Non-White Concerns in Personnel and Guidance, 4*(1), 5-15.

Buber, M. (1970). *I and Thou* (transl. W. Haufman). Edinburgh: T & T Clark (original work published 1923).

Buchheimer, A. & Balogh, S.C. (1961). *The Counseling Relationship*. Chicago: Science Research Associates.

Buergenthal, T. (1979). Codification and implementation of international human rights. In A.H. Henken (ed.), *Human Dignity: The Internationalization of Human Rights* (pp. 15-23). Copublishers: Aspen Institute for Humanistic Studies, New York; Oceana Publications; New York; Netherlands: Sijthoff & Noordhoff.

Buhrmann, M.V. (1977). Xhosa diviners as psychotherapists. *Psychotherapeia, 21,* 17-20.

Buhrmann, M.V. (1983). Community health and traditional healers. *Psychotherapeia, 9,* 15-18.

Bulhan, H.A. (1980). Dynamics of cultural in-betweenity: An empirical study. *International Journal of Psychology, 152,* 105-121.

Bulhan, H.A. (1985). *Franz Fanon and the Psychology of Oppression.* New York: Plenum Press.

Bulhan, H.A. (1990). Afro-centric psychology: Perspective and practice. In L. Nicholas & S. Cooper (eds.), *Psychology and Apartheid* (pp. 66-75). Johannesburg: Vision Publications.

Bulhan, H.A. (1993). Imperialism in studies of the psyche: A critique of African psychological research. In L. Milolos (ed.), *Psychology and Oppression: Critiques and Proposals*, pp. 1-34. Johannesburg: Skottavile Publishers.

Burman, E. (1990). Differing with deconstruction: A feminist critique. In I. Parker & J. Shotter (eds.), *Deconstructing Social Psychology* (pp. 208-220). New York: Routledge.

Burman, E., & Parker, I. (1993). Introduction—Discourse analysis: The turn to the text. In E. Burman & I Parker (eds.), *Discourse Analytic Research* (pp. 1-13). London: Routledge.

Business Day, March 1990.

Burt, K. & Oaksford, M. (1999). Qualitative methods: Beyond beliefs and desires. *The Psychologist, 12* (7), 332-335.

Calia, V.F. (1966). The culturally deprived client: Re-formulation of the counselor's role. *Journal of Counseling Psychology, 13,* 100-105.

Carkhuff, R.R. (1969). *Helping and Human Relations.* New York: Holt, Rinehart & Winston.

Carlton, E. 1977). *Ideology and Social Order.* London: Routledge & Kegan Paul.

Carpenter, C. (1987). *Introduction to South African Constitutional Law.* Durban: Butterworths.

Carpy, D. (1989). Tolerating the countertransference: A mutative process. *International Journal of Psychoanalysis. 70,* 287-294.

Carrim, N. (2000). Critical antiracism and problems in self-articulated forms of identities. *Race, Ethnicity and Education, 3*(1), 25-44.

Carter, J.H. (1994). Racism's impact on mental health. *Journal of the National Medical Association, 86,* 543-547.

Carter, R.T. (1995). *The Influence of Race and Racial Identity in Psychotherapy: Toward a Racially Inclusive Model.* New York: John Wiley & Son.

Carter, R.T. & Helms, J.E. (1990). White racial identity attitudes and cultural values. In J.E. Helms (ed.), *Black and White Racial Identity: Theory, Research, and Practice* (pp. 105-118). Westport, CT: Greenwood Press.

Casas, J.J. (1984). Policy training and research in counseling psychology: The racial/ethnic minority perspective. In S. Brown & R. Lent (eds.), *Handbook of Counseling Psychology* (pp. 785-831). New York: John Wiley.

Castel, R., Castel, F., & Lovell, A. (eds.) (1982). *The Psychiatric Society.* Columbia University Press.

Cavill, S. (2000). From prisoner to president. *The Psychologist, 13*(1), 14-15.

Caylef, S.E. (1986). Ethical issues in counseling gender, race, and culturally distinct groups. *Journal of Counseling and Development, 64,* 345-347.

Celani, D.P. (1993). The therapist's approach to the inner world of the borderline. In *The Treatment of the Borderline Patient: Applying Fairbairn's Object Relations Theory in a Clinical Setting.* Madison: International Universities Press Inc.

Chambers, J.C. (1992). Triad Training: A method for teaching basic counseling skills to chemical dependency counselors. Ph.D. Dissertation. University of South Dakota.

Charmaz, G. (1995). Grounded theory. In J.A. Smith, R. Harré & L. Van Langenhove (eds.), *Rethinking Methods in Psychology*, London, Thousand Oaks, CA and New Delhi: Sage.

Chunn, J.C., Dunston, P., & Ross-Sheriff, F. (eds.), (1983). *Mental Health and People of Color.* Washington D.C.: Howard.

Citron, A. (1969) *The Rightness of Whiteness: World of a White Child in a Segregated Society* (pamphlet). Detroit: Ohio Regional Educational Lab (available from P.A.C.T., Detroit).

Clarkson, P. (1990). A multiplicity of psychotherapeutic relationships. *British Journal of Psychotherapy, 7*(2), 148-163.

Cleaver, E. (1968). *Soul on Ice.* New York: Dell.

Cloete, N., & Pillay, S. (1988). Professional neutrality: In the service of the clients and/or the professionals. *Psychology in Society. 9,* 44-65.

Cloete, N., Pillay, S. & Swart, A. (1986). The pro-active counselor: Is neutrality possible? Paper presented at the Annual Conference of the Society for Student Counseling in South Africa, Johannesburg.

Cobbs, P. (1972). Ethnotherapy. *Intellectual Digest, 2,* 26-28.

Cock, J. (1980). *Maids and Madams.* Johannesburg: Ravan Press.

Cohen, D (1989). Soviet Psychiatry: *Politics and Mental Health in the USSR Today.* London: Paladin.

Cole, J. (1996). *Beyond Prejudice: Teaching Tools: A Triad Model Approach for the reduction of prejudicial behavior.* Ellensburg, WA: Growing Images.

Cole, J. & Pilisuk, M. (1976). Differences in the provision of mental health services by race. *American Journal of Orthopsychiatry, 46,* 510-525.

Coltart, N. (1995). A Philosopher and his Mind. In *The Pathology and Precocity of Self Sufficiency.* London: Sage.

Comas-Diaz, L. & Padilla, A. (1990). Countertransference in working with victims of political repression. *American Journal of Orthopsychiatry, 60,* 125-134.

Combrink-Graham (1987). Invitation to kiss: Diagnosing ecosystemically *Psychotherapy, 24*(3), 505-515.

Cooper, M. & Rowan, J. (1999). Introduction: Self-plurality—the one and the many. In J. Rowan & M. Cooper (eds.), *The Plural Self. Multiplicity in Everyday Life* (pp. 1-10). Sage.

Cooper, S. (1973). A look at the effect of racism on clinical work. *Social Casework, 54* (2), 76-84.

Cooper, S. & Nicholas, L. (1990). Preface. In L.J. Nicholas & S. Cooper (eds.), *Psychology and Apartheid.* Johannesburg: Vision Publication.

Cooper, S., Nicholas, L.J., Seedat, M., & Statmann, J.M. (1990). Psychology and Apartheid: the struggle for psychology in South Africa. In L.J. Nicholas & S. Cooper (eds.), *Psychology and Apartheid.* Johannesburg: Vision Publications.

Coppard, L.E. & Steinwachs, B.J. (1970). Guidelines for community action. In E.L. Perry (ed.), *The White Problem.* Philadelphia: United Presbyterian Church.

Coyle, A. (1995). Discourse analysis. In G.M. Breakwell, S. Hammond & C. Fife-Shaw (eds.), *Research Methods in Psychology* (pp. 243-258). Thousand Oaks, CA; London; & New Delhi: Sage.

Crosby, F., Bromley, S., & Saxe, L. (1980). Recent unobtrusive studies of black and white discrimination and prejudice: A literature review. *Psychological Bulletin, 87,* 546-563.

Danieli, Y. (1985). The treatment and prevention of long-term effects and intergenerational transmissions of victimization: A lesson from Holocaust survivors and their children. In C. Figley (ed.), *Trauma and Its Wake* (pp. 295-313). New York: Brunner/Mazel.

Dawes, A. (1985). Politics and mental health: The position of clinical psychology in South Africa. *South African Journal of Psychology,15,* 55-56.

Dawes, A. (1986). Educating South African mental health and social service professionals: Considerations for change in training and research. Apartheid and Mental Health: OASSA National Conference 17-18 May 1986. Organization for Appropriate Social Services in South Africa.

Day, A.T. (1983). Childbearing practices in the Appalachian culture. *Frontier Nursing Science Quarterly Bulletin, 59,* 1-7.

Dean, E., Hartmann, P., & Katzen, M. (1983). *History in Black and White.* Paris: Unesco.

De Groof, J. & Malherbe, R. (1997). Introduction. In J. De Groof & E.F.J. Malherbe (eds.), *Human Rights in South African Education: From the Constitutional Drawing Board to the Chalkboard.* (pp. 25-34). The Netherlands: Uitgeverij Acco.

Delamont, S. (1991). *Fieldwork in Educational Settings: Methods, Pitfalls, and Perspectives.* London: Falmer Press.

Dell, P.F. (1982). Beyond homeostasis: Toward a concept of coherence. *Family Process, 21,* 21-41.

Dell, P.F. (1985). Understanding Bateson and Maturana: Toward a biological foundation for the social sciences. *Journal of Marital and Family Therapy, 11*(1), 1-20.

Denzin, N.K. & Lincoln, Y.S. (1994). *Handbook of Qualitative Research*: Thousand Oaks, CA; London; & New Delhi: Sage.

Derrida, J. (1978). *Writing and Difference.* London: Routledge & Kegan Paul.

Derrida, J. (1983). Letter to a Japanese friend. In D. Wood & R. Bernaseoni (eds.), *Derrida and Difference.* Evanston, IL: Northwestern University Press.

De Shazer, S. (1982). Some conceptual distinctions are more useful than others. *Family Process, 21,* 71-84.

De Shazer, S. (1984). The death of resistance. *Family Process, 23,* 11-17.

Devenish, G.E. (1998). *A Commentary on the South African Constitution.* Durban, Butterworths.

De Villiers, S.A. (1971). *Robben Island.* Cape Town: Struik.

Dey, I. (1993). *Qualitative Data Analysis: A User-Friendly Guide for Social Scientists.* London and New York: Routledge.

Dhadphale, M., Ellison, R. & Griffin, L. (1983). The frequency of psychiatric disorders among patients attending semi-urban and rural general out-patient clinics in Kenya. *British Journal of Psychiatry, 142,* 379-383.

Dinstein,Y. (1976). Collective human rights of people and minorities. *International and Comparative Law Quarterly, 25,* 102-120.

Disco, C. (1979). Critical theory as ideology of the new class. *Theory and Society,* 159-211.

Dlamini, C., (1997). The relationship between human rights and education. In J. De Groof & E.F.J. Malherbe. *Human Rights in South African Education: From the Constitutional Drawing Board to the Chalkboard* (pp. 39-52). The Netherlands: Uitgeverij Acco.

Draguns, J.G. (1981). Cross-cultural counseling and psychotherapy: History, issues, current status. In A.J. Marsella and P.B. Pedersen (eds.), *Cross-Cultural Counseling and Psychotherapy* (pp. 3-27). New York: Pergamon Press.

Draguns, J.G. (1989). Dilemmas and choices in cross-cultural counseling: The universal versus the culturally distinctive. In P.B. Pedersen, J.G. Draguns, W.J. Lonner, & J.E. Trimble (eds.), *Counseling Across Cultures* (pp. 3-22). Honolulu: University of Hawaii.

Drower,S. (2002). Conceptualizing social work in a changed South Africa. *International Social Work, 45(1),* 7-20.

Du Bois, W.E.B. (1965, original in 1903). Souls of Black folk. In J.H. Franklin (ed.), *Three Negro Classics.* New York: Avon.

Du Bois, W.E.B. (1969). *The Souls of Black Folk.* New York: Signet.

Dubow, S. (1987). Race, civilization, and culture. In S. Marks & S.T. Trapido (eds.), *The Politics of Race, Class, and Nationalism in Twentieth Century South Africa.* London: Longman.

Duckitt, J. (1992). *The Social Psychology of Prejudice.* New York: Praeger.

Dugard, J. (1998). Public international law. In Chaskelson et al. (eds.), *Constitutional Law of South Africa.* (pp. 13.1-13.11). Cape Town: Juta.

Duncan, N. (1998). Special issue: Black scholarship. Challenging academic racism in South African psychology. In L. Schlebusch (ed.), *South Africa Beyond Transition: Psychological Well-being.* Proceedings of the 3rd Annual Congress of the Psychological Society in South Africa.

Duncan, N. & Rock, B. (1995). South African children and public violence: Quantifying the damage. *Psychology Resource Centre Occasional Publication Series, No 19,* University of the Western Cape.

Duncan, N., Seedat, M., Van Niekerk, A., de la Rey, C., Gobodo-Madikizela,P., Simbayi, L.C., Bhana, A. (1997). Black scholarship: Doing something active and positive about academic racism. *South African Journal of Psychology, 27*(4), 201-213.

Du Preez, J.J. (1983). Africana Afrikaner: *Master Symbols in South African School Textbooks.* Alberton: Librarius.

Durant. T. & Sparrow. K. (1997). Race and class consciousness among lower-and-middle class blacks. *Journal of Black Studies. 27*(3): 334-351.

Durrheim, K. (2000). Racism in the private and public spheres. *Research Review, Eastern Seaboard Association of Tertiary Institutions, 15*, 3-7.

Durrheim, K. & Mokeki, S. (1997). Race and relevance: A content analysis of the South African Journal of Psychology. *The South African Journal of Psychology, 27*(4), 206-213.

Du Toit, A. (1983). The chosen people: The myth of the Calvinist origins of Afrikaner nationalism and racial ideology. *American Historical Review, 88*, 920-952.

Eagle, G. (1998). *Male Crime Victim: The Social and Personal Construction of Meaning in Response to Traumatogenic Events.* Ph.D. Dissertation. Johannesburg; University of the Witwatersrand.

Easton, D. (1971). *The Political System.* New York: Knopf.

Edelstein, I, Weber, V., and Pillay, Y. (1997). The role of the private sector. In D. Foster, M. Freeman, & Y. Pillay (eds.), *Mental Health Policy Issues for South Africa* (pp. 132-142). MASA: Multimedia Publications.

Edler, J. (1974). White on White: An antiracism manual for White educators in the process of becoming. Ph.D. Dissertation. University of Massachussets.

Egan, G. (1986). *The Skilled Helper: A Systematic Approach to Effective Healing.* Monterey, CA: Brooks/Cole.

Eisenberg, L. (1995). The social construction of the human brain. *American Journal of Psychiatry, 152*, 1563-1575.

Elkaim, M. (1981). Nonequilibrium, chance, and change in family therapy. *Journal of Marital and Family Therapy,* Summer.

Ellis, A. (1962). *Reason and Emotion in Psychotherapy.* New York: Lyle Stuart.

Epstein, L. (1979). Countertransference with borderline patients. In L. Epstein & A. Feiner (eds.), *Countertransference: The Therapist's Contribution to the Therapeutic Situation.* New York: Jason Aronson.

Erikson, E.H. (1958). The nature of clinical evidence. *Daedalus, 87*, (4), 65-87.

Erikson, E. (1963). *Childhood and Society.* New York: Norton.

Erikson, E. (1964). *Insight and Responsibility.* New York: Norton.

Essed, P. (1987). *Academic Racism.* Amsterdam: CRES.

Essed, P. (1991). *Understanding Everyday Racism: An Interdisciplinary Theory.* Newbury Park, London, & Delhi: Sage.

Etzioni, (1991). *A Responsive Society.* San Francisco: Jossey-Bass.

Etzioni, (1993). *The Spirit of Community.* New York: Touchstone.

Fanon, F.O. (1986 a). *Black Skin, White Masks.* London: Pluto Press.

Fernando, S. (1986). Depression in ethnic minorities. In J.L. Cox (ed.), *Transcultural Psychiatry.* London: Croom Helm.

Fernando, S. (1988). *Race and Culture in Psychiatry.* London: Croom Helm.

Fernando, S. (1991). *Mental Health, Race, and Culture.* London: Macmillan.

Financial Mail, 3 June 1988.

Finchelescu, G. & Nyawose, G. (1998). Talking about language: Zulu students' views on language in the new South Africa. *South African Journal of Psychology, 28* (2), 53-61.

Fireside, H. (1979). *Soviet Psychoprisons.* New York: W. W. Norton & Company.

Firestone, R.W. (1997a). *Combating Destructive Thought Processes: Voice Therapy and Separation Theory.* Thousand Oaks, CA: Sage.

Firestone, R.W. (1997b). *Suicide and the Inner Voice: Risk Assessment, Treatment, and Case Management.* Thousand Oaks, CA: Sage

Fisch, R., Weakland, J.H., & Segal, L. (1982). *The Tactics of Change*. San Francisco: Jossey-Bass Publishers.

Flisher, A.J., Skinner, D., Lazarus, S., & Louw, J. (1993). Organizing mental health workers on the basis of politics and service: The case of the Organization of Appropriate Social Services in South Africa (pp. 236-245). In L.J. Nicholas (ed.), *Psychology and Oppression: Critiques and Proposals*. Johannesburg: Skottaville.

Fontana, A. & Frey, J.H. (1994). Interviewing: The art of science. In N.K. Denzin & Y.S. Lincoln (eds.), *Handbook of Qualitative Research* (pp. 361-376). Thousand Oaks, CA; London; & New Delhi: Sage.

Foster, D. (1986). The development of social orientation in children: A review of South African research. In S. Burman & P. Reynolds (eds.), *Growing Up in a Divided Society: The Contexts of Childhood in South Africa*. Johannesburg: Ravan Press.

Foster. D (1991). Race and racism in South African psychology. *South African Journal of Psychology, 21* (4); 203-210.

Foster, D. (1993). The mark of oppression? Racism and psychology considered. In L.J. Nicholas (ed.), *Psychology and Oppression: Critiques and Proposals* (pp. 128-141). Johannesburg: Skottaville.

Foster, D. & Louw-Potgieter, J. (1992). *Social Psychology in South Africa*. Johannesburg: Lexicon Publishers.

Foster, D., Nicholas, L. & Dawes, A. (1993). A reply to Raubenheimer. *The Psychologist,* April, pp. 172-174.

Foucault, M. (1965). *Madness and Civilization: A History of Insanity in the Age of Reason.* New York: Vintage Books.

Foucault, M. (1972). *The Archeology of Knowledge*. London: Tavistock.

Foucault, M. (1976). *Mental Illness and Psychology*. New York: Harper Colophon Books.

Foucault, M. (1977). *Discipline and Punish: The Birth of the Prison.* New York: Vintage Books.

Foucault, M. (1988). Technologies of the self. In L.H.Martin, H.Gutman and P.H. Hutton (eds.), *Technologies of the Self.* London: Tavistock.

Foucault, M. (1990). *Michel Foucault: Interview and Other Writings, 1977-1984.* L. Kritzman (ed.), New York: Routledge.

Fox, D.R. (1993). The autonomy—community balance and the equity law distinction: Anarchy's task for psychological jurisprudence. *Behavioral Sciences and the Law,* 11, 97-109.

Frankenberg, R. (1993). *White Women, Race Matters: The Social Construction of Whiteness.* Minneapolis: University of Minnesota Press.

Frazer, E. & Lacey, N. (1993). *The Politics in Community: A Feminist Critique of the Liberal-Communitarian Debate.* Toronto, Ontario, Canada: University of Toronto Press.

Freeman, M. (1991). Mental Health for all—moving beyond rhetoric. *South African Journal of Psychology, 21(3),* 141-147.

Freeman, M. (1992). Providing mental health care for all in South Africa—Structure and strategy. Paper No. 24, Centre for Health Policy, University of the Witwatersrand.

Freeman, M. & Pillay, Y. (1997). Mental health policy—plans and finding. In D. Foster, M. Freeman & Y. Pillay (eds.), *Mental Health Policy Issues for South Africa.* Medical Association of South Africa.

Freud, S. (1910). The future prospects of psycho-analytic therapy. *Standard Edition, 11,* 139-151. London: Hogarth.

Fuqua, D.R., Newman, J.L., Andersen, M.W., & Johnson, A.W. (1986). *Psychological Reports 38,* 163-172.

Gaertner, S.L. & Dovidio, J.F. (1986). The aversive form of racism. In J.F. Dovidio & S.L. Guertner (eds.), *Prejudice, Discrimination and Racism* (pp. 61-89). Orlando, FL: Academic Press.

Galton, F. (1869). *Hereditary Genius: An Inquiry into Its Laws and Consequences.* London: Macmillan.

Gardner, L.K. (1971). The therapeutic relationship under varying conditions of race. *Psychotherapy: Theory, Research, and Practice, 8,* 78-87.

Gergen, K.J. (1994). *Realities and Relationships: Soundings in Social Construction.* Cambridge, MA: Harvard University Press.

Gergen, K.J. & Gergen, M.M. (1988). Narrative and the self as relationship. *Advances in Experimental Social Psychology, 21,* 17-56.

Gibson, K., Sandenbergh, R., & Swartz (2001). Becoming a community clinical psychologist: Integration of community and clinical practices in psychologists' training. *South African Journal of Psychology, 31*(1), 29-35.

Giddens, A. (1990). *Sociology.* Oxford: Polity Press.

Gillis, L.S., Koch, A., & Joyi, M. (1989). Improving compliance in Xhosa psychiatric patients. *South African Medical Journal, 72,* 205-208.

Glaser, B.G. & Strauss, A.L. (1967). *The Discovery of Grounded Theory: Strategies for Qualitative Research.* Chicago, IL: Aldine.

Gobodo, P. (1990). Notions about culture in understanding black psychopathology: Are we trying to raise the dead? *South African Journal of Psychology, 20,* 93-98.

Gobodo-Madikizela, P. (1997). Healing the racial divide? Personal reflections on the Truth and Reconciliation Commission. *South African Journal of Psychology 27*(4), 271-272.

Goffmann, E. (1968). *Assylums.* Hanmondsworth: Penguin.

Goldberg, D.T. (1994). *Racist Culture: Philosophy and the Politics of Meaning.* Oxford: Blackwell.

Goodwin, J. (1984). *Cry Amandla! South African Women and the Question of Power.* Johannesburg: Africana Publishing House.

Gordon, J. (1965). Project cause: The federal antipoverty program and some implications of sub-professional training. *American Psychologist, 20,* 333-343.

Grotstein (1997) "Internal objects" or "chimerical monsters?" The demonic "third forms" of the internal world. *The Journal of Analytical Psychology, 42,* 47-80.

Greenberg, J.R. & Mitchell, S.A. (1983). *Object Relations in Psychoanalytic Theory.* Cambridge: Harvard University Press.

Greene, B.A. (1985). Consideration in the treatment of black patients by white therapists. *Psychotherapy,* 22, 293-389.

Greenson, R.R. (1967). *The Technique and Practice of Psychoanalysis.* Vol. 1. New York: International Universities Press.

Griffith, M.S. (1977). The influence of race on the psychotherapeutic relationship. *Psychiatry, 40,* 27-40.

Gumede, M. (1990). *Traditional Healers.* South Africa: Skotaville.

Habermas, J. (1990). Justice and solidarity: On the discussion concerning "stage 6." In M. Kelly (ed.), *Hermeneutics and Critical Theory in Ethics and Politics* (pp. 21-42). Cambridge, MA: MIT Press.

Habermas, J. (1990). *Moral Consciousness and Communicative Action.* Cambridge, MA: MIT Press.

Hall, G.S. (1905). The Negro in Africa and America. *Pedagogical Seminary, 12,* 350-368.

Halleck, S.L. (1971). Therapy is the handmaiden of the status quo. *Psychology Today.* pp. 30-34, 98-100.

Hamilton, N.G. (1992). The containing function and the analyst's projective identification. In N.G. Hamilton (ed.), *From Inner Resources: New Directions in Object Relations Psychotherapy.* (pp. 163-180). Northvale, N.J.: Jason Aronson.

Hamilton, N.G. (ed.), (1992). *From Inner Resources: New Directions in Object Relations Psychotherapy.* Northvale, N.J.: Jason Aronson.

Hammond-Tooke, D. (1989). *Rituals and Medicine.* Johannesburg: Donker Press.

Harris, C. (1997). The moral repudiation of apartheid in Jewish classical sources. *Jewish Affairs,* Autumn 1997, pp. 58-59.

Harrison, D. (1981). *The White Tribe of Africa.* University of California Press.

Hartman, W. (1995). *Ego State Therapy with Sexually Traumatized Children.* Pretoria: Kagiso.

Hauck, P. (1990). *How to Stand Up for Yourself.* London: Sheldon Press.

Hayes, G. (1986). Intervening with the political psyche. In *Apartheid and Mental Health. OASSA National Conference, 17-18 May 1986.* Organisation for Appropriate Social Services in South Africa.

Haysom, N., Strous, M., & Vogelman, L. (1990). The mad Mrs. Rochester revisited: The involuntary confinement of the mentally ill in South Africa. *South African Journal of Human Rights, 6*(3), 341-362.

Haysom, N., Strous, M., & Vogelman, L. (1992). The mad Mrs. Rochester revisited. The involuntary confinement of the mentally ill in South Africa. *Psychology in Society, 16,* 6-31.

Health Professions Council of South Africa (1999). *The Professional Board for Psychology Ethical Code of Professional Conduct.* HPCSA.

Heather, N. (1976). *Radical Perspectives in Psychology.* London: Methuen.

Heimann, P. (1950). On countertransference. *International Journal of Psychoanalysis, 31,* 81-84.

Heimann, P. (1960). Countertransference. *British Journal of Medical Psychology, 33,* 9-15.

Heine, R.W. (1950). The Negro patient in psychotherapy. *Journal of Clinical Psychology, 6,* 373-376.

Heller, K. & Monahan, J. (1977). *Psychology and Community Change.* Chicago, IL: Dorsey Press.

Helms, J.E. (1984). Toward an explanation of the influence of race in the counseling process: A Black-White model. *The Counseling Psychologist, 12,* 153-165.

Helms, J.E. (1986). Expanding racial identity theory to cover counseling process. *Journal of Counseling Psychology, 33*(1), 62-64.

Helms, J.E. (1990). Review of racial identity terminology. In J.E. Helms (ed.). *Black and White Racial Identity: Theory, Research, and Practice* (pp. 1-8). New York: Greenwood Press.

Helms, J.E. (1994). Racial identity and "racial" constructs. In E.J. Trickett, R. Watts, & D. Birman (eds.), *Human Diversity* (pp. 285-311). San Francisco: Jossey-Bass.

Helms, J.E. & Carter, R.T. (1991). Relationships of White and Black racial identity attitudes and demographic similarity to counselor preferences. *Journal of Counseling Psychology, 38*(4), 446-457.

Helms, J.E. & Piper, R.E. (1994). Implications of racial identity theory for vocational psychology. *Journal of Vocational Behavior, 44,* 124-138.

Henderson, P. (1976). Class structure and the concept of intelligence. In R. Dales & G. Esland (eds.), Schooling *and Capitalism.* London: Routledge & Kegan Paul.

Hendriks, A. & Toebes, B. (1998). Towards a universal definition of the right to health? *Medicine and Law, 17,* 319-332.

Henriques, J., Hollway, W., Urwin, C., & Walkerdine, V. (1984). *Changing the Subject: Psychology, Social Regulation and Subjectivity.* London: Methuen.

Henwood, K.L. (1996). Qualitative inquiry: Perspectives, methods, and psychology. In J.T.E. Richardson (ed.), *Handbook of Qualitative Research Methods for Psychology and the Social Sciences* (pp. 25-42). Leicester: BPS Books.

Henwood, K.L. & Pidgeon, N.F. (1992). Qualitative research and psychological theorizing. *British Journal of Psychology, 83,* 97-111.

Henwood, K. & Nicholson, P. (1995). Qualitative research. *The Psychologist, March 1995,* 109-110.

Henwood, K. & Pidgeon, N. (1995a). Grounded theory and psychological research. *The Psychologist, 8,* 115-118.

Henwood, K.L. & Pidgeon, N.F. (1995b). Theory, grounding and reflexivity: Another route to constructivist psychology? Unpublished manuscript. Brunel University and Birkbeck College.

Hermans, H.J.M. (1996). Voicing the self: From information processing to dialogical interchange. *Psychological Bulletin, 119*(1), 31-50.

Hermans, H.J.M & Kempen, H.J.G. (1993). *The Dialogical Self: Meaning as Movement*. London and San Diego, CA.: Academic Press.

Hermans, H.J.M., Rijks, T.I., & Kempen, H.J.G. (1993). Imaginal dialogues in the self: Theory and method. *Journal of Personality, 61* (2), 207-236.

Hernandez, A.G. & Kerr, B.A. (1985). *Evaluating the Triad Model and Traditional Cross-Cultural Counselor Training*. Presented at the 93rd Annual Convention of the American Psychological Association in Los Angeles, CA.

Hernstein, R.J. (1994). *The Bell Curve: Intelligence and Class Structure in American Life*. New York: Free Press.

Herr, E.L. (1987). Cultural diversity from an international perspective. *Journal of Multicultural Counseling and Development, 15*, 99-110.

Herzog, A. (1984). On multiple personality: Comments on diagnosis, etiology and treatment. *International Journal of Clinical and Experimental Hypnosis*, 32: 210-221.

Hickson, J., Christie, G. & Shmukler, D. (1990). A pilot study of world view of Black and White South African adolescent pupils: Implications for cross-cultural counselling. *South African Journal of Psychology, 20* (3), 170-177.

Hickson, J. & Kriegler, S. (1996). *Multicultural Counseling in a Divided and Traumatized Society: The Meaning of Childhood and Adolescence in South Africa*. Westport, CT & London: Greenwood Press.

Hickson, J. & Strous, M. (1993). The plight of South African women domestics: Providing the ultra-exploited with psychologically empowering mental health services. *Journal of Black Studies, 24*(1), 109-122.

Hines, A. & Pedersen, P. (1980). The cultural grid: Matching social system variables and cultural perspectives. *Asian Pacific Training Development Journal, 1*(1), 5-11.

Ho, M.K. (1987). *Family Therapy with Ethnic Minorities*. Newbury Park, CA: Sage.

Hoffman, L. (1981). *Foundation of Family Therapy*. New York: Basic Books.

Hoffman, L. (1982). A coevolutionary framework for systemic family therapy. *Australian Journal of Family Therapy, 4*, 9-21.

Hoffman, L. (1985). Beyond power and control: Toward a "second order" family systems therapy. *Family Systems Medicine, 3*(4), 381-396.

Holdstock, L. (1981a). Indigenous healing in South Africa and the person oriented approach of Carl Rogess. *Curare, 4*, 31-46.

Holdstock, T.L. (1981b). Psychology in South Africa belongs to the colonial era: Arrogance or ignorance? *South African Journal of Psychology, 11*, 123-129.

Hollway, W. (1989). *Subjectivity and Method in Psychology: Gender, Meaning, and Science*. London: Sage.

Hooks, B. (1996). *Killing Rage: Ending Racism*. London: Penguin Books.

Hopa, M., & Simbayi, L.C., & Du Toit, C.D. (1998). Perceptions on integration of traditional and western healing in the new South Africa. *South African Journal of Psychology, 28*(1), 8-14.

Horowitz (1982). Court legislated reform: Viable approach or proper victory? In R. Castel, F. Castel, & A. Lovell (eds.), *The Psychiatric Society*. New York: Columbia University Press.

Hountondji, P.J. (1983). *African Philosophy: Myth and Reality*. London: Hutchinson University Library for Africa.

Howe, M.J.A. (1998). Can I.Q. change? *The Psychologist, February*, pp. 69-72.

Ibanez, I. & Iniquez, L. (eds.), (1997). *Critical Social Psychology*. London: Sage.

Ibrahim, F.A. & Arrendondo, P.M. (1986). Ethical standards for cross-cultural counseling preparation, practice, assessment, and research. *Journal of Counseling and Development, 64*, 349-351.

Ingleby, D. (1981). *Critical Psychiatry*. Harmondsworth: Penguin.

Irvin, R. & Pedersen, P. (1995). The internal dialogue of culturally different clients: An application of the Triad Model. *Journal of Multicultural Counseling and Development*.

Ivey, A. (1980). *Counseling and Psychotherapy: Connections and Applications*. New York: Prentice Hall.

Ivey, A.E. & Authier, J. (1978). *Microcounseling: Innovations in Interviewing Training*. Springfield IL: Charles C. Thomas.

Ivey, G. (1986). Elements of a critical psychology. *Psychology in Society, 5*, 4-27.

Ivey, G. (1992). Countertransference pathology in South African psychotherapy. *Psychoanalytic Psychotherapy in South Africa*, Spring, 1992, 31-45.

Jackson, A.M. (1973). Psychotherapy: Factors associated with the race of the therapist. *Psychotherapy: Theory, Research and Practice, 10*(3), 273-277.

Jackson, M.A. (1996). Stereotype reversal in counselor training. Dissertation Proposal, Stanford University.

Jacoby, R. (1975). *Social Amnesia*. Sussex: Harvester Press.

Janis, I.C. (1982). *Counseling on Personal Decisions: Theory and Research on Short Term Helping Relationships*. Yale University Press.

Jenkins, J.H. & Valiente, M. (1994). Bodily transactions of the passions: El calor among Salvadoran refugees. In T.J. Csordas (ed.), *Embodiment and Experience: The Existential Ground of Culture and Self* (pp. 163-182). Cambridge University Press.

Jensen, A.R. (1969). How much can we boost IQ and scholastic achievement? *Harvard Educational Review, 39*(1), 1-123.

Johnson, F.A. (1986). Ethnicity and international rules in counseling: Rules in counseling and psychotherapy: Some basic considerations. In A.J. Marsella & P.B. Pedersen (eds.), *Crosscultural Counseling and Psychotherapy* (pp. 63-83). New York: Pergamon Press.

Johnson, J.L. & Wildersen, F.B. (1969). The institute for research on the social and emotional development of Afro-American children. Manuscript Proposal. Syracuse, N.Y.

Johnson, S.D. (1990). Toward clarifying culture, race, and ethnicity in the context of multicultural counseling. *Journal of Multicultural Counseling and Development, 18*(1), 41-50.

Johnston, H. (1995). A methodology for frame analysis: From discourse to cognitive sclemata. In H. Johnston & B. Klandermans (eds.), *Social Movements and Culture, Social Movements, Protest and Contention*, Vol. 4. (pp. 217-247). University of Minnesota Press.

Jones, A. & Seagull, A.A. (1977). Dimensions of the relationship between the Black client and White therapist. *American Psychologist, 32;* 850-855.

Jones, J.M. (1992). Understanding the mental health consequences of race: Contributions of basic social psychological processes. In D.N. Ruble, P.R. Costanzo & M.E. Oliveri (eds.), *The Social Psychology of Mental Health: Basic Mechanisms and Applications* (pp. 199-240). New York: Guilford Press.

Jones, J.M. (1997). *Prejudice and Racism* (2nd ed.) New York: McGraw-Hill.

Jordaan, W. & Jordaan, J. (1985). *Man in Context*. Johannesburg: McGraw-Hill.

Jordan G. & Weedon, C. (1995). *Cultural Politics: Class, Gender, Race, and the Postmodern World*. Oxford: Basil Blackwell.

Jordan, W.D. (1968). *White Over Black*. University of North Carolina Press.

Jung, C.G. (1930). Your Negroid and Indian behavior. *Forum, 83*, 193-199.

Kagan, N. (1964). Three dimensions of counselor encapsulation. *Journal of Counseling Psychology, 11*, 361-365.

Kamin, L. (1974). *The Science and Politics of IQ*. London: John Wiley.

Kaplan, B.H. (1971). *Blue Ridge: An Appalachian community in transition*. Morgantown, WV: Office of Research and Development, Appalachian Center, West Virginia University.

Kaplan, H. & Sadock, B. (1985). *Comprehensive Textbook of Psychiatry*. London: Williams & Wilkins.

Katz, J.H. (1982). *White Awareness: Handbook for AntiRacism Training*. Norman: University of Oklahoma Press.

Keeney, B.P. (1979). Ecosystemic epistemology: An alternative paradigm for diagnosis. *Family Process, 18*(2), 117-129.

Keightly, R. (1992). International human rights norms in a new South Africa. *South African Journal on Human Rights, 8;* 171-187.

Kelley, A.W. (in press). Client secret keeping in outpatient therapy. *Journal of Counseling Psychology.*

Kentridge, J. (1996). Equality. In Chaskelson et al. (eds.), *Constitutional Law of South Africa* (pp. 14.1-14.46). Cape Town: Juta.

Kernberg, O.F. (1974). Further contributions to the treatment of narcissistic personalities. *International Journal of Psychoanalysis, 55,* 215-240.

Kincheloe, J.L. & McLaren, P.L. (1998). Rethinking initial theory and qualitative research. In N.K. Denzin & Y.S. Lincoln (eds.), *Handbook of Qualitative Research* (pp. 138-157). Thousand Oaks, CA; London; & New Delhi: Sage.

Kinder, D.R. (1986). The continuing American dilemma: White resistance to racial change 40 years after Myrdal. *Journal of Social Issues, 4,* 151-171.

Kinder, D.K. & Sears, D.O. (1981). Prejudice and politics: Symbolic racism versus racist threats to the good life. *Journal of Personality and Social Psychology, 40,* 414-431.

King, E. (1996). The use of the self in qualitative research. In J.T.E. Richardson (ed.), *Handbook of Qualitative Research Methods for Psychology and the Social Sciences* (pp. 175-188). Leicester: BPS Books.

Klein, M. (1948). *The Psychoanalysis of Children.* London: Hogarth Press.

Kleinman, A. (1986). *Social Origins of Distressed Disease: Depression, Neuroasthenia and Pain in Modern China.* New Haven, CT and London: Yale University Press.

Knowles, L. & Prewitt, K. (eds.), (1969). *Institutional Racism in America.* Englewood Cliffs, NJ: Prentice-Hall.

Kohut, H. (1972). Thoughts on narcissism and narcissistic rage. *The Psychoanalytic Study of the Child, 27,* 360-400.

Kohut, H. (1977). *The Restoration of the Self.* New York: International Universities Press.

Korenberg & Korenberg (1981). Psychiatry: The lost horizon. *Legal Medicine, 81.*

Korf, G. & Schoeman, J.B. (1996). Applicability of Milstones' DIB-C model in the South African context. *South African Journal of Psychology, 26*(4), 212-220.

Korman, M. (1974). National conference on levels and patterns of professional training in psychology: Major themes. *American Psychology, 29,* 301-313.

Kottler, A. (1990). South Africa: Psychology's dilemma of multiple discourses. *Psychology in Society, 13,* 27-36.

Kovel, J. (1970). *White Racism: A Psychohistory.* New York: Pantheon.

Kovel, J. (1982). Values, interests, and psychotherapy. *American Journal of Psychoanalysis, 42*(2), 109-119.

Kriegler, S. (1993). Options and direction for psychology within a framework for mental health services in South Africa. *South African Journal of Psychology, 23*(2), 64-70.

Kroeber, A.L. & Kluckhohn, C. (1952). *Culture: A Critical Review of Concepts and Definitions.* New York: Vintage Books.

Kuzel, A.J. (1992). Sampling in qualitative inquiry. In B.F. Crabtree & W.L. Miller (eds.), *Research Methods for Primary Care* (pp. 33-44). London: Sage.

La Frambois, T.D. & Foster, S.L. (1989). Ethics in multicultural counseling. In P.B. Pedersen, J.G. Draguns, W. J. Lomer, & J.E. Trimble (eds.), *Counseling Across Cultures* (pp. 115-136). Honolulu: University of Hawaii.

La Grange, A.J. (1962). Die agtergrond en die vernaamste taakstellings van SIRSA. Monografie No. 1 van die Sielkundige Instituut van die Republiek van Suide Afrika.

Lambert, M.J. (1986). Implications of psychotherapy outcome research for eclectic psychotherapy. In J.C. Nocross (ed.), *Handbook of Eclectic Psychotherapy* (pp. 436-462). New York: Brunner/Mazel.

Lambley, P. (1980). *The Psychology of Apartheid.* London: Seker & Warburg.

Landrine, H. & Klonoff, E.A. (1996). The schedule of racist events: A measure of racial discrimination and a study of its negative physical and mental health consequences. *Journal of Black Psychology, 22,* 144-168.

Landy, R. (1993). *Persona and Performance.* London: Jesica Kingsley Publishers.

Lange, A.J. & Jacubowski, P. (1976). *Responsible Assertive Behavior: Cognitive/Behavioral Procedures for Trainers*. Champaign, IL: Research Press.

Lau, A. (1984). Transcultural issues in family therapy. *Journal of Family Therapy, 6,* 91-112.

Layder, D. (1993). Grounded theory and field research. In D. Layder *New Strategies in Social Research: An Introduction and Guide* (pp. 38-50). Cambridge: Polity Press.

Lazarus, S. (1985). The role and responsibility of the psychologist in the South African context. Survey of psychologists' opinions. Paper delivered at the Third National Congress of the Psychological Association of South Africa, Pretoria.

Lea, S.J. (1996). That ism on the end makes it nasty: Talking about race with young White South Africans. *South African Journal of Psychology, 26,* 183-190.

Lewin, K. (1969). Quasi-stationary social equilibria and the problem of permanent change. In W.G. Bennis, K.D Benne, & R.Chin (eds.), *The Planning of Change*. New York: Holt, Rinehart & Winston.

Lewis, L. & Appleby, L. (1988). Personality disorders: The patients psychiatrists dislike. *British Journal of Psychiatry, 153,* 44-49.

Lewis-Fernández, R. & Kleinman, A. (1995). Cultural psychiatry: Theoretical clinical and research issues. *The Psychiatric Clinics of North America, 18,* 433-448.

Lind, J.E. (1913). The dream as a simple wish fulfillment in the Negro. *The Psychoanalytical Review, 1,* 295-300.

Little, M. (1951). Countertransference and the patient's response to it. *International Journal of Psychoanalysis, 32,* 32-40.

Littlewood, R. & Lipsedge, M. (1997). *Aliens and Alienists: Ethnic Minorities and Psychiatry.* London & New York: Routledge.

Locke, D. & Lewis, S.O. (1969). Racism encountered in counseling. *Counselor Education and Supervision, 9,* 49-60.

Loo, C. (1980a). *Bicultural Contextualizer Model for Cultural Sensitivity in Counseling: Transcript. Harmful Assumptions.* Santa Cruz. CA: Chinatown Research Center and the University of California.

Loo, C. (1980b). *Bicultural Contextualiser Model for Cultural Sensitivity in Counseling: Transcript. Understanding Ethnic Identity.* Santa Cruz, CA: Chinatown Research Centre and the University of California.

Louw, A. du P. (1983). Democracy. In D.J. Van Vuuren & D.J. Kriek (eds.), *Political Alternatives for Southern Africa.* Durban: Butterworths.

Louw, J. (2002). Psychology, history, and society. *South African Journal of Psychology, 32* (1), 1-8.

Luckhurst, P. (1985). Resistance and the new epistemology. *Journal of Strategic and Systemic Therapies, 4,* 9-21.

Luria, A. (1961) *The Role of Speech in the Regulation of Normal and Abnormal Behaviors.* New York: Liveright.

Maakhe, N.P. (1994). Dismantling the Tower of Babel: In search of a new language policy for South Africa. In R. Fardon & G. Furniss (eds.), *African Languages, Development and the State* (pp. 111-121). London: Routledge.

MacCrone, I.D. (1937). *Race Attitudes in South Africa: Historical, Experimental and Psychological Studies.* London: Oxford University Press.

MacDonell, D. (1986). *Theories of Discourse: An Introduction.* Oxford: Basil Blackwell.

Mackay and Fanning (1994). *Self-esteem.* Oakland,CA: New Harbinger.

Macleod, C. & Durrheim, K. (in press). Racializing teenage pregnancy: "Culture" and "tradition" in the South African scientific literature. *Ethnic and Racial Studies.*

Magubane, B. (1979). *The Political Economy of Race and Class in South Africa.* New York: Monthly Review Press.

Mahoney, M. (1974). *Cognitive and Behavior Modification.* Cambridge, MA: Ballinger Publishing Co.

Mahrer, A.R. (1996). *The Complete Guide to Experiential Psychotherapy.* New York: Wiley.

Majodina, M. & Attah-Johnson, F. (1983). Standardized assessment of depressive disorders (SADD) in Ghana. *British Journal of Psychiatry, 143,* 442-446.

Malan, D.H. (1979). *Individual Psychotherapy and the Science of Psychodynamics.* Durban: Butterworths.

Malherbe E.F.J. & Rautenbach, I.M. (1996). Preface. In I.M. Rautenbach & E.F.J. Malherbe, *Constitutional Law.* Durban: Butterworth Publishers.

Manganyi, N.C. (1991). *Treachery and Innocence: Psychology and Racial Difference in South Africa.* Johannesburg: Ravan Press.

Maranhão, T. (1984). Family therapy and anthropology. *Culture, Medicine and Society, 8,* 255-279.

Marsella, A.J. & Pedersen, P.B. (1981). *Cross-Cultural Counseling and Psychotherapy.* New York: Pergamon Press.

Martindale, C. (1980) Subselves: The internal representations of situational and personal dispositions. In L. Wheeler (ed.), *Review of Personality and Social Psychology,* Vol. 1. Beverly Hills, CA: Sage.

Maturana, H. (1978). The biology of language: The epistemology of reality. In G. Miller & E. Lenneberg (eds.), *Psychology and the Biology of Language and Thought.* New York: Academic Press.

Mays, V.M. (1985). The black American and psychotherapy: A dilemma. *Psychotherapy, 22*(2), 379-388.

Mbeki, T. (1998). *Africa: The Time Has Come.* Cape Town: Tafelberg.

McConahay, J.B. (1986). Modern racism, ambivalence, and the modern racism scale. In J.F. Dovidio & S.L. Gaertner (eds.), *Prejudice, Discrimination, and Racism* (pp. 91-125). San Diego: Academic Press.

McDougall, W. (1908). *Social Psychology.* New York.

McGoldrick, M. (1982). Ethnicity and family therapy: An overview. In M. McGoldrick, J.K. Pearce & J. Giordano (eds.), *Ethnicity and Family Therapy.* New York: Guilford Press.

McKall, R.B. (1986). *Fundamental Statistics for Behavioral Science* (4th ed.). Harcourt Bruce Jovanovich.

McNamee, S. & Gergen, K.J. (1992). *Therapy as Social Construction.* Newbury Park, CA: Sage.

Mead, G.H. (1934). *Mind, Self, and Society* (C.W. Morris, ed.). Chicago, IL: University of Chicago Press.

Mead, G.H. (1982). *The individual and the social self: Unpublished work of George Herbert Mead.* D.L. Miller (ed.), University of Chicago Press.

Meichenbaum, D.H. (1974). *Cognitive Behavior Modification.* Marristown, N.J: General Learning Press.

Meichenbaum, D.H. (1975). Self-instructional methods (how to do it). In A. Goldstein & F. Kanfer (eds.), *Helping People Change: Methods and Materials.* New York: Pergamon Press.

Meichenbaum, D.H. (1977). *Cognitive Behavior Modification: An Intergrative Approach.* New York: Plenum Press.

Miles, R. (1989). *Racism.* London: Routledge.

Milner, D. (1997). Racism and childhood identity. *The Psychologist: Bulletin of the British Psychological Society, 10*(3), 123-125.

Mkhize, N.J. & Frizelle, K. (2000). Hermeneutic-dialogical approaches to career development: An exploration. *South African Journal of Psychology, 30*(3), 1-8.

Mohutsioa-Makhudu, Y. (1989). The psychological effects of apartheid on the mental health of Black South African women domestics. *Journal of Multicultural Counseling and Development, 17,* 134-142.

Moll, I. (2002). African psychology: Myth and reality. *South African Journal of Psychology, 32*(1), 9-16.

Montagu, A. (1964). *Man's Most Dangerous Myth: The Fallacy of Race* (4th ed.). Cleveland: World.

Moore, R. (1973). A rationale, description, and analysis of a racism awareness program for White teachers. Ed. D. Diss. University of Massachussets.

Moosa, F. (1992). Countertransference in trauma work in South Africa: For better or worse. *South African Journal of Psychology, 22,* 126-133.

Morin, A. (1993). Self talk and self awareness: On the nature of the relation. *Journal of Mind and Behavior, 14*(3), 223-224.

Mulvey, A. (1981) community psychology and feminism: Tensions and commonalities. *Journal of Community Psychology, 16,* 70-83.

Mureinik, E. (1994). A bridge to where? Introducing the interim bill of rights. *South African Journal on Human Rights, 10,* 31-48.

Murgatroyd, W. (1995). Application of the Triad Model in teaching counseling skills in providing immediate supervision. Unpublished Manuscript. University of New Orleans.

Nagan & Atkins (2002). Conflict resolution and democratic transformation: Confronting the shameful past-prescribing a humane future. *The South African Law Journal.*

Naidoo, A. (2000). Book review: Multiculturalism as a fourth force, by Paul Pedersen. *South African Journal of Psychology, 30* (4), 52-53.

Neimeyer, G.J., Fukayama, M.A., Bingham, R.P., Hall, L.E., & Mussenden, M.E. (1986). Training cross-cultural counselors: A comparison of the pro and anticounselor Triad Models. *Journal of Counseling and Development, 64,* 437-439.

Nell, V. (1990). One world, one psychology: "Relevance" and ethnopsychology. *South African Journal of Psychology, 20(3),* 129-140.

Nell, V. (1993). Structural blocks to a liberatory psychology in South Africa: Medical politics, guild consciousness, and the clinical delusion. In L.J. Nicholas (ed.), *Psychology and Oppression: Critiques and Proposals* (pp. 212-235). Johannesburg: Skottaville Publishers.

Nicholas, L.J. (1990). The response of South African professional psychology associations to apartheid. *Journal of the History of the Behavioral Sciences, 25,* 58-63.

Nicholas, L.J. (1993). The response of student counselors in South Africa to racism in higher education. In L.J. Nicholas (ed.), *Psychology and Oppression: Critiques and Proposals.* Johannesburg: Skottaville Publishers.

Nkomo, M., Mkwanazi-Twala, Z., & Carrim, N. (1995). The long shadow of apartheid ideology: The use of open schools in South Africa. In B.P. Bowser (ed.), *Racism and AntiRacism in World Perspective,* pp. 261-284. Thousand Oaks, CA and London: Sage.

Nortier, S.E. & Theron, W.H. (1998). Acculturation in post-apartheid South Africa: A time of healing or a time of identity confusion and loss? In L. Schlebusch (ed.), *South Africa Beyond Transition: Psychological Well-Being.* Proceedings of the 3rd Annual Congress of the Psychological Society of South Africa (pp. 230-233). Psyssa.

Nutt-Williams, E. & Hill, C.E. (1996). The relationship between self-talk and therapy process variables for novice therapists. *Journal of Counseling Psychology, 43,* (2) 170-177.

O'Connell, D.C. & Kowal, S. (1995). Basic principles of transcription. In J.A. Smith, R. Harré & L. Van Langenhove. *Rethinking Methods in Psychology.* (pp. 93-105). Thousand Oaks, CA; London; & New Delhi: Sage.

Odejide, A., Oyewunmi, L., & Ohaeri, J. (1989). Psychiatry in Africa: An overview. *American Journal of Psychiatry, 146,* 708-715.

O'Hanlon, W.H. (1992). Not systemic, not strategic: Still useless after all these years. *Journal of Strategic and Systemic Therapies, 10,* 105-110.

O'Malley, M. (1914). Psychoses in the colored race. *Journal of Insanity, 71,* 309-336.

Orley, J. & Wing, J. (1979). Psychiatric disorders in two African villages. *Archives of General Psychiatry, 36,* 513-520.

Owusu-Bempah, K. & Howitt, D. (1999). Even their soul is defective. *The Psychologist, 12*(3), 126-130.

Packer, H.L. (1964). Two models of the criminal process. *University of Pennsylvania Law Review, 118.*

Padilla, A.M., Ruiz, R. & Alvarez, R. (1975). Community mental health services for the Spanish-speaking-surnamed population. *American Psychologist, 30,* 892-905.

Padilla, E., Boxley, R. & Wagner, N. (1972). The desegregation of clinical psychology training. Paper presented at the meeting of the American Psychological Association, Honolulu.

Pagels, E. (1979). The roots and origins of human rights. In A.H. Henkin (ed.), *Human Dignity: The Internationalization of Human Rights.* (pp. 1-8). Copublishers: Aspen Institute for Humanistic Studies, New York; Oceana Publications, New York; and Sijthoff and Noordhoff, Netherlands.

Painter, D.W. & Theron, W.H. (1998). Identity, difference, and embodiment: On the ethical and political implications of theorizing social identity in the South African context. In L. Schlebusch (ed.), *South Africa Beyond Transition: Psychological Well-Being* (pp. 238-242). Proceedings of the 3rd Annual Congress of the Psychological Society of South Africa. Pretoria: PSYSSA.

Papp, P. (1977). The family that had all the answers. In Papp, P. (ed.), *Family Therapy: Full Length Case Studies.* New York: Gardner Press.

Parham. T.A. & Helms, J.E. (1985). Relation of racial identity attitudes to self-actualization and affective states of Black students. *Journal of Counseling Psychology, 32,* 431-440.

Paris, J. (1998). Psychotherapy for the personality disorders: Working with traits. *Bulletin of the Menninger Clinic, 62*(3), 287-297.

Parker, I. (1992) *Discourse Dynamics: Critical Analysis for Social and Individual Psychology.* London: Routledge.

Parker, I. (1999). Deconstruction and psychotherapy. In I. Parker (ed.), *Deconstructing Psychotherapy* (pp. 1-18). Thousand Oaks, CA; London; & New Delhi: Sage.

Parker, I. & Shotter, J. (eds.), (1990). *Deconstructing Social Psychology.* London: Routledge.

Parry, A. (1984). Maturanation in Milan: Recent developments in systemic therapy. *Journal of Strategic and Systemic Therapies, 3*(1), 35-42.

Patel, M. (1998). Black therapists—White clients: An exploration of experiences in cross-cultural therapy. *Clinical Psychology Forum.*

Patel, N., Bennett, E., Dennis, M., Dosanjh, N., Mahtani, A., Miller, A., & Nadirshaw, Z. (2000). *Clinical Psychology, 'Race,' and Culture: A Training Manual.* Leicester: BPS Books (The British Psychological Society).

Patton, M.Q. (1980). *Quantitative Evaluation Methods.* London: Sage.

Pedersen, P. (1976a). A model for training mental health workers in cross-cultural counseling. In J. Westermeyer (ed.), *Anthropology and Mental Health.* New York: Basic Books.

Pedersen, P.B. (1976b). Counseling clients from other cultures: Two training designs. In M.K. Asante, E. Newmark & C.A. Blake (eds.), *Handbook of Intercultural Communication.* California: Sage.

Pedersen, P. (1977). The Triad Model of cross-cultural counselor training. *Personnel and Guidance Journal, 56,* 94-100.

Pedersen, P.B. (1978). Four dimensions of cross-cultural skills in counselor training. *Personnel and Guidance Journal, 57,* 480-484.

Pedersen, P. (1982). The intercultural context of counseling and therapy. In A. Marsella & G. White (eds.), *Cultural Conceptions of Mental Health and Therapy,* 333-358. Dordrecht, Holland: D Reidel.

Pedersen, P.B. (1983). Intercultural training of mental health providers. In D. Landis & R.W. Brislin (eds.), *Handbook of Intercultural Training.* Vol. 2. New York: Pergamon Press.

Pedersen, P.B. (1985). Triad counseling. In R. Corsini (ed.), *Innovative Psychotherapies.* (pp. 840-854) New York: Wiley.

Pedersen, P. (1988). *A Handbook for Developing Multicultural Awareness.* Virginia: American Association for Counseling and Development.

Pedersen, P.B. (1991). Multiculturalism as a generic approach to counseling. *Journal of Counseling and Development, 70,* 6-12.

Pedersen, P.B. (1997). *Culture-Centered Counseling Interventions: Striving for Accuracy.* Thousand Oaks, CA; London; & New Delhi: Sage.

Pedersen, P.B. (1999). *Multiculturalism as a Fourth Force.* Philadelphia, PA: Brunner/Mazel.

Pedersen, P.B. (2000a). *A Handbook for Developing Multicultural Awareness.* (3rd ed.) Virginia: American Association for Counseling and Development.

Pedersen, P.B. (2000b). *Hidden Messages in Culture-Centered Counseling: A Triad Training Model.* Thousand Oaks, CA; London; & New Delhi: Thousand Oaks, CA; London; & New Delhi: Sage.

Pedersen, P.B. & Ivey, A. (1993). *Culture Centered Counseling and Interviewing Skills: A Practical Guide.* Westport, CT: Praeger.

Pedersen, P. & Leong, F.L. (1997). Counseling in an international context. *The Counseling Psychologist, 25(*1), 117-120.

Pedersen, P. & Pedersen, A. (1989). The cultural grid: A complicated and dynamic approach to multicultural counseling. *Counseling Psychology Quarterly, 2,* 133-141.

Peebles-Kleiger, M. (1989). Using countertransference in the hypnosis of trauma victims: A model for turning hazard into healing. *American Journal of Psychotherapy, 43,* 518-530.

Penn, P. (1982). Circular questioning. *Family Process, 21,* 267-280.

Penn, P. & Frankfurt, M. (1994). Creating a participant text: Writing, multiple voices, narrative multiplicity. *Family Process, 33*(3), 217-231.

Perkel, A. (1988). Towards a model for a South African clinical psychology. *Psychology in Society, 10,* 53-75.

Perkins, D.D., & Zimmerman, M.A. (1995). Empowerment theory, research, and application. *American Journal of Community Psychology, 23,* 569-580.

Perls, F.S. (1976). *The Gestalt Approach.* Palo Alto: Bantam Books.

Peterson, B. (1999). Identity in the round: Between Whiteness and the African renaissance. *Thinking Through the African Rennaissance Seminar Series.* The Graduate School for the Humanities and Social Sciences, University of the Witwatersrand.

Pidgeon, N. (1996). Grounded Theory: Theoretical background. In J.T. Richardson (ed.), *Handbook of Qualitative Research Methods for Psychology and the Social Sciences.* Leicester: BPS Books.

Pidgeon, N. & Henwood, K. (1996). Grounded theory: Practical implementation. In J.T. Richardson (ed.), *Handbook of Qualitative Research Methods for Psychology and the Society Sciences.* Leicester: BPS Books.

Pilgrim, D. (1997). *Psychotherapy and Society.* London: Sage.

Pillay, Y.G. & Petersen, I. (1996). Current practice patterns of clinical and counseling psychologists and their attitudes to transforming mental health policies in South Africa. *South African Journal of Psychology, 26*(2), 76-81.

Pinderhughes, C.A. (1973). Racism and psychotherapy. In C. Willie, B. Kramer & B. Brown (eds.), *Racism and Mental Health.* Pittsburgh: University of Pittsburgh Press.

Pinderhughes, E. (1984). Teaching empathy: Ethnicity, race, and power at the cross-cultural treatment intervention. *American Journal of Social Psychiatry, 4*(1), 5-12.

Pines, D. (1986). Working with women survivors of the holocaust: Affective experiences in transference and countertransference. *International Journal of Psychoanalysis, 67,* 295-307.

Platzky, L. & Walker, C. (1985). *The Surplus People.* Johannesburg: Ravan Press.

Pollack, J. & Levy, S. (1989). Countertransference and failure to report child abuse and neglect. *Child Abuse and Neglect, 13,* 515-522.

Ponterotto, J.G. & Pedersen, P.B. (1993). *Preventing Prejudice: A Guide for Counselors and Educators.* Thousand Oaks, CA; London; & New Delhi: Sage.

Poortinga, Y.H. (1990). Towards a conceptualization of culture for psychology. *Cross-Cultural Psychology Bulletin, 24*(3), 2-10.

Potter, J. & Wetherell, M. (1992). *Discourse and Social Psychology: Beyond Attitudes and Behavior.* London: Sage.

Powis, P. (1989). Resistance: Who's resisting whom? In J. Mason & J. Rubenstein (eds.), *Family Therapy in South Africa Today.* Congella, Natal: South African Institute of Marital and Family Therapy.

Preston-Whyte, E.M. (1976). Race attitudes and behavior: The case of domestic employment in White South African homes. *African Studies, 35*, 75-89.

Prigogine, I. (1978). Time, structure and fluctuations. *Science, 201,* 777-795.

Prilleltensky, I. (1997). Values, assumptions, and practices: Assessing the moral implications of psychological discourse and action. *American Psychologist, 52*(5), 517-535.

Prudhomme, C. & Musto, D.F. (1973). Historical perspectives on mental health and racism in the United States. In C.V. Willie, B.M. Kramer, & B.S. Brown (eds.), *Racism and Mental Health*. University of Pittsburgh Press.

Psychological Association of South Africa (1989). *Mental Health in South Africa: Report by the Council Committee: Mental Health.*

Rack, P. (1982). *Race, Culture and Mental Disorder.* London: Tavistock Publications.

Racker, H. (1957). The meanings and uses of countertransference. *Psychoanalytic Quarterly, 26*, 303-357.

Radford, E.J. & Rigby, C.J. (1986). An open systems model for the analysis of psychology in a changing socio-political environment. Paper presented at the Fourth National Conference of the Psychological Association of South Africa.

Rappaport, J. (1977). *Community Psychology: Values, Research, and Action.* New York: Holt, Rinehart & Winston.

Rappaport, J. (1981). In praise of paradox: A social policy of empowerment over prevention. *American Journal Of Community Psychology, 9 (1),* 1-23.

Rappaport, J. (1987). Terms of empowerment/exemplars prevention: Toward the theory for community psychology. *American Journal of Community Psychology, 15 (2),* 121-147.

Raubenheimer, I. Van W. (1993). Psychology in South Africa. *The Psychologist, April 1993,* pp. 169-171.

Reich, A. (1951). On countertransference. *International Journal of Psychoanalysis. 32,* 25-31.

Reicher, S. (1999). Differences, self-image and the individual. *The Psychologist, 12*(3), 131-133.

Reoch, R. (1994). Editor's viewpoint. In *Human Rights: The New Consensus.* London: Regency Press.

Rhoodie, N.J. (1983). *Value Consensus as a Prerequisite for Consociational Federalism in Southern Africa: Principles and Perspectives.* Pretoria: Butterworths.

Richards, G. (1988). The case of psychology and "race". *The Psychologist, 11*(4), 179-181.

Richards, G. (1997). *"Race," Racism, and Psychology: Towards a Reflexive History.* London and New York: Routledge.

Richards, G. (1998). The case of psychology and "race." *The Psychologist, 11*(4), 179-181.

Richardson, L. (1994). Writing: A method of inquiry. In N.K. Denzin & Y.S Lincoln (eds.), *Handbook of Qualitative Research* (pp. 516-592). Thousand Oaks, CA; London; and New Delhi: Sage.

Richardson, T.Q. & Molinaro, K.L. (1996). White counselor self-awareness: A prerequisite for multicultural competence. *Journal of Counseling and Development, 74*(3), 238-242.

Richter, L. (1994). Economic stress and its influence on the family and caretaking patterns. In A. Dawes & D. Donald (eds.), *Childhood and Adversity* (pp. 28-50). Cape Town: David Phillip.

Richter, L.M., Griesel, R.D., Durrheim, K., Wilson, M., Surrendorff, N. & Asafo-Agyei, L. (1998). Employment opportunities for psychology graduates in South Africa: A contemporary Analysis. *South African Journal of Psychology, 28*(1), 1-7.

Ridley, C.R. (1989). Racism in counseling as an aversive behavioral process. In P.B. Pedersen, J.G. Draguns, W.J. Lonner & J.E. Trimble (eds.), *Counseling across Cultures* (3rd ed.) (pp. 55-77). University of Hawaii Press.

Ridley, C.R. (1995). *Overcoming Unintentional Racism in Counseling and Therapy: Practitioner's Guide to Intentional Intervention.* Thousand Oaks, CA: Sage.

Rogers, C.R. (1961). *On Becoming a Person.* Boston: Houghton-Mifflin.

Rogers, C.R. (ed.), (1967). *The Therapeutic Relationship and Its Impact.* Madison, WI: University of Wisconsin Press.

Rose, N. (1988). Calculable minds and manageable individuals. *History of the Human Sciences, 1,* 179-200.

Rosenau, P.J. (1992). *Post-Modernism and the Social Sciences: Insights and Intrusions.* Princeton, NJ: Princeton University Press.

Rousseau, J.J. (1762). *Du Contract Social.* (1963 trans.). *The Social Contract and Discourses,* trans. and intro. by G.D.H. Cole. London and New York: Everyman's Library.

Rowan, J. (1990). *Subpersonalities: The People Inside Us.* London: Routledge.

Rowan, J., & Cooper, M. (1999). Introduction: Self-plurality—the one and the many. In J. Rowan & M. Cooper (eds.), *The Plural Self. Multiplicity in Everyday Life* (pp. 1-10). Thousand Oaks, CA; London; & New Delhi: Sage.

Rumble, S., Swartz, L., Parry, C., & Zwarenstein, M. (1996). Prevalence of psychiatric morbidity in the adult population of a rural South African village. *Psychological Medicine, 26,* 997-1007.

Rushton, J.P. (1988). Race differences in behavior: A review and evolutionary analysis. *Journal of Personality and Individual Differences, 9,* 1009-1024.

Rwegellera, G. & Mambwe, C. (1977). Diagnostic classification of first-ever admissions to Chainama Hills Hospital, Lusaka, Zambia. *British Journal of Psychiatry, 130,* 573-580.

Sabshin, M. et al. (1970). Dimensions of Institutional racism in psychiatry. *American Journal of Psychiatry, 127,* 787-793.

Sachs, A. (1985). Towards the reconstruction of South Africa. *Journal of South African Studies 12,* 49.

Sager, C.J. et al. (1972). Black patient-White therapist. *American Journal of Orthopsychiatry, 42,* 415-423.

Sandler, J., Holder, A., & Dare, C. (1970). Basic psychoanalytic concepts: IV Countertransference. *British Journal of Psychiatry, 117,* 83-88.

Sarbin, T.R. (1993). Foreword. In H.J.M. Hermans & H.J.G. Kempen. *The Dialogical Self: Meaning and Movement.* (pp. xii-xv). New York: Academic Press.

Satir, V. (1964). *Conjoint Family Therapy.* Palo Alto, CA: Science and Behavior Books.

Schlemmer, L. (1996). The nemesis of race: A case for redoubled concern. *Frontiers of Freedom.* South African Institute of Race Relations. Third Quarter, 21-24.

Schoeman, J.B. (1989). Psigopatologie by tradisionele swart Suid Afrikaners. In D.A. Louw (ed.), *Suid Afrikaanse Handboek van Abnormale Gedrag* (pp. 448-470). Johannesburg: Southern.

Schwandt, T.A. (1998). Constructivist, interpretevist approaches to human inquiry. In N.K. Denzin & Y.S. Lincoln. *Handbook of Qualitative Research.* (pp. 118-137). Thousand Oaks, CA; London; & New Delhi: Sage.

Schwartz, R. (1987). Our multiple selves, *Family Therapy Networker, 11(2),* 25-31.

Schwartz, R. (1995). *The Internal Family Systems Therapy.* New York: Guilford.

Seares, D. (1988). Symbolic racism. In D.A. Katz & D.A. Taylor (eds.), *Eliminating Racism: Profiles in Controversy* (pp. 53-84). New York: Plenum.

Searles, H. (1965). The informational value of the supervisor's emotional experiences. In *Collected Papers on Schizophrenia and Related Subjects.* London: The Hogarth Press.

Seedat, M. (1990). Programs, trends, and silences in South African Psychology, 1983-1988. In L. Nicholas & S. Cooper (eds.), *Psychology and Apartheid* (pp. 22-49). Johannesburg: Vision Publications.

Seedat, M. (1997). The quest for liberatory psychology. *South African Journal of Psychology, 27(4),* 261-270.

Seedat, M. (1998). A characterization of South African Psychology (1948-1988): The impact of exclusionary ideology. *South African Journal of Psychology, 28(2),* 74-84.

Seedat, M. & Nell, V. (1990). Third world or one world: Mysticism, pragmatism, and pain in family therapy in South Africa. *South African Journal of Psychology, 20(3),* 141-149.

Seedat, M. & Nell, V. (1992). Conflicting value systems in the introduction of psychological services in a South African Primary Health Care System. *South African Journal of Psychology, 22(4),* 185-193.

Shapiro, S.B. (1976). *The Selves Inside You*. Berkeley, CA: Explorations Institute.

Sherrard, C. (1997). Never mind the bath water, keep hold of the baby! Qualitative research. *The Psychologist: Bulletin of the British Psychological Society, 10*(4), 161-162.

Shivji, I.G. (1999). Constructing a new rights regime: Promises, problems, and prospects. *Social and Legal Studies, 8*(2), 253-276.

Shockley, W. (1971). Negro IQ deficit: Failure of a "malicious coincidence" model warrants new research proposals. *Review of Educational Research, 41*(3), 227-248.

Shotter, J. (1997). Dialogical realities: The ordinary, the everyday, and other strange new worlds. *Journal for the Theory of Social Behavior, 27*, 345-57.

Shuey, A.M. (1966). *The Testing of Negro Intelligence*. New York: Social Science Press.

Shweder, R.A. (1990). Cultural psychology—What is it? In J.W. Stigler, R.A. Shweder, & G. Herdt (eds.), *Cultural Psychology: Essays on Comparative Human Development* (pp.1-43). New York: Cambridge University Press.

Sieghart, P. (1988). An introduction to the international convention on human rights: Paper proposed for the Commonwealth Secretariat. *Human Rights Unit Occasional Paper*. London: Commonwealth Secretariat.

Sifrin, G., Friedman, S. & Bellar, D. (1997). Can reconciliation take root in post-apartheid South African society? A Jewish view on the process. *Jewish Affairs*, Autumn 1997, pp. 63-68.

Simkin, J.S. & Yontef, G.M. (1984). Gestalt therapy. In R.J. Corsini (ed.), *Current Psychotherapies* (pp. 279-319). Itasca, IL: Peacock.

Sluzki, C.E. (1983). Process, structure, and world views: Toward an integrated view of systemic models in family therapy. *Family Process, 22*, 469-476.

Smith, D. (1980). The impact of world-views on professional life-styling. *Personnel and Guidance Journal, 58*, 584-587.

Sokolov, A.N. (1972). *Inner Speech and Thought*. New York: Plenum Press.

South African Institute of Race Relations. (1987). *1987 Race Relations Survey*. Johannesburg: South African Institute of Race Relations.

South African Institute of Race Relations (1992). *Annual Survey 1991-1992*. Johannesburg: South African Institute of Race Relations.

Spero, M. & Mester, R. (1988). Countertransference envy toward the religious patient. *The American Journal of Psychoanalysis, 48*, 43-55.

Stampp, K.M. (1956). *The Peculiar Institution: Slavery in the Ante-Bellum South*. New York: Knopf.

Statistics for South Africa (2000). Retrieved October 2002 from World Wide Web: http//geohive.com/cd/sf.php

Steinberg, D. (n.d.) *Racism in America: Definition and Analysis*. (Pamphlet, available through P.A.C.T., Detroit).

Stern, E. (1987). The race script of the counselor: Concepts from transactional analysis. *International Journal for the Advancement of Counseling, 10*, 35-43.

Stevens, G. (1998). "Racialized" discourses: Understanding perceptions of threat in post-apartheid South Africa. *South African Journal of Psychology, 28*(4), 204-214.

Stevenson, C. & Cooper, N. (1997). Qualitative and quantitative research. *The Psychologist: The Bulletin of the British Psychological Society, 10*(4), 159-160.

Stone, H. and Winkelman, S. (1989). *Embracing Ourselves: The Voice Dialogue Manual*. Mill Valley, CA: Nataraj Publishing.

Straker, G. (1987). Unpublished lecture to the post graduate training course. Integrative Psychotherapy Association (South Africa), at the University of the Witwatersrand, Johannesburg.

Straker, G. (1989). Emotional abuse of children in South Africa. Unpublished manuscript.

Straker, G. (1994). Integrating African and Western healing practices in South Africa. *American Journal of Psychotherapy, 48*(3), 455-467.

Strauss, L. (1975). What is political philosophy? *Journal of Politics, 19*(3), 343-368.

Strauss, S.A. (1981). Le syndrome du bon Dieu. (Cited in *Living*, 1988).

Strauss, A.L. & Corbin, J. (1990). *Basics for Qualitative Research: Grounded Theory Procedures and Techniques.* Newbury Park, California: Sage.

Strauss, A.L. & Corbin, J. (1994). Grounded theory methodology: An overview. In N.K. Denzin & Y.S. Lincoln (eds.), *Handbook of Qualitative Research* (pp. 273-285). Thousand Oaks, CA; London; & New Delhi: Sage.

Strebel, A., Msomi, N., & Stacey, M. (1999). A gender and racial epidemiological profile of public psychiatric hospitals in the Western Cape. *South African Journal of Psychiatry, 29,* 53-61.

Strous, M. (1992). Use of the Triad Model in training family therapists for work with diverse South African Groups. Unpublished Diss. University of the Witwatersrand.

Strous, M. (1997). Therapists' inner dialogue in interracial counseling contexts. Unpublished research proposal. University of the Witwatersrand.

Strous, M. & Eagle, G. (in process). Anticlient and Proclient Positions in Interracial Therapy.

Strous, M. Skuy, M. & Hickson, J. (1993). Perceptions of the Triad Model's efficacy in training family counselors for diverse South African groups. *International Journal for the Advancement of Counseling, 16,* 307-318.

Sturgeon, S (2002). Developing Cultural Awareness In Human Service Professionals: A Personal Journey. *Social work/Maatskaplike Werk,* 38(2), 173-181.

Strydom, H.A. (1998). Minority rights protection: Implementing international standards. *South African Journal on Human Rights, 3*(14), 373-387.

Sue, D.W. (1977). Counseling the culturally different: A conceptual analysis. *Personnel and Guidance Journal, 55,* 422-426

Sue, D.W. (1979a). *Annual evaluation report on developing interculturally skilled counselors.* NIMH training project. Honolulu, Hawaii.

Sue, D.W. (1979b). Eliminating cultural oppression in counseling: Toward a general therapy. *Journal of Counseling Psychology, 25,* 419-428.

Sue, D.W. (1981). *Counseling the Culturally Different: Theory and Practice.* New York: Wiley.

Sue, D.W., Arredondo, P., & McDavis, R.J. (1992). Multicultural counseling competencies and standards: A call to the profession. *Journal of Counseling and Development, 20,* 477-486.

Sue, D.W., Ivey A.E., & Pedersen, P.B. (1996). *Multicultural Counseling Theory.* Pacific Grove, CA: Brooks/Cole.

Sue, D.W. & Sue, D. (1977). Barriers to effective cross-cultural counseling. *Journal of Counseling Psychology, 24,* 420-429.

Sue, D.W. & Sue, D. (1990). *Counseling the Culturally Different: Theory and Practice* (2nd ed.). New York: John Wiley.

Sue, S. & Zane, N. (1987). The role of culture and cultural techniques in psychotherapy: A critique and reformulation. *American Psychologist, 62*(1), V, 37-45.

Swartz, L. (1987). Transcultural psychiatry in South Africa. Part II. *Transcultural Psychiatric Research Review, 24,* 5-30.

Swartz, L. (1988). Some comments on the draft ethical code for South African clinical psychologists. *South African Journal of Psychology, 18*(1), 17-20.

Swartz, L. (1991). The reproduction of racism in South African mental health care. *South African Journal of Psychology, 21*(4), 240-246.

Swartz, L. (1998). *Culture and Mental: A Southern African View.* Cape Town: Oxford University Press.

Swartz, L. (1999). Multiculturalism and mental health in a changing South Africa. In P. Pedersen (ed.), *Multiculturalism as a Fourth Force.* Philadelphia, PA: Brunner/Mazel.

Swartz, L., Drennan, G., & Crawford, A. (1997). Changing language policy in mental health services: A matter of interpretation. In D. Foster, M. Freeman, & Y. Pillay (eds.), *Mental Health Policy Issues for South Africa* (pp. 166-180). Cape Town: MASA Multimedia.

Swartz, L. & Foster, D. (1984). Images of culture and mental illness: South African psychiatric approaches. *Social Dynamics, 10*(1), 17-25.

Swartz, L., Gibson, K., & Swartz, S. (1990). State violence in South Africa and the development of a progressive psychology. In N.C. Manganyi & A. du Toit (eds.), *Political Violence and the Struggle in South Africa* (pp. 234-264). London: Macmillan.

Swartz, R.M. & Garamoni, G.L. (1989). Cognitive balance and psychopathology: Evaluation of an information processing model of positive and negative states of mind. *General Psychology Review, 9,* 271-294.

Swartz, S. (1995). Colonizing the insane: Courses of insanity in the Cape, 1891-1920. *History of the Human Sciences, 8*(4), 39-57.

Swartz, S. (1999). Using psychodynamic formulations in South African clinical settings. *South African Journal of Psychology, 29*(1), 42-48.

Swartz, S., Dowdall, T., & Swartz, L. (1986). Clinical psychology and the 1985 crisis in Cape Town. *Psychology in Society, 5,* 131-138.

Szazs, T. (1970). *Ideology and Insanity.* New York: Doubleday.

Tajfel, H. (1978). *The Social Psychology of Minorities.* London: Minorities Rights Group.

Terman, L.M. (1916). *The Measurement of Intelligence.* Boston: Houghton-Mifflin.

Terry, R. (1970). *For Whites Only.* Grand Rapids, MI: Eerdmans, 1970.

Thabede, D.G. (1991). The relevance of traditional healers in the provision of mental health services. *Social Work Journal, 2,* 11-14.

The British Psychological Association. (1993). *Code of Conduct, Ethical Principles and Guidelines* (1993). Leicester: BPS.

The Professional Board for Psychology. (2002) *Ethical Code of Professional Conduct.* Health Professions Council of South Africa.

The Star, various issues.

The Weekly Mail, various issues.

Thomas, A. (1962). Pseudo-transference reactions due to cultural stereotyping. *American Journal of Orthopsychiatry, 32*(5), 894-900.

Thomas, A. & Sillen, S. (1972). *Racism and Psychiatry.* New York: Brunner/Mazel.

Tobias, P.T. (1972). *The Meaning of Race* (2nd ed.). South African Institute of Race Relations.

Tomm, K. (1989). Externalizing the problem and internalizing personal agency. *Journal of Strategic and Systemic Therapies, 8*(1), 54-69.

Trepagnier, B. (1994). The politics of White and Black bodies. *Feminism and Psychology, 4,* 199-205.

Tribe (1988). *American Constitutional Law.*

Truax, C.B. & Carkhuff, R.R. (1965). Client and therapist transparency in the psychotherapeutic encounter. *Journal of Counseling Psychology, 12,* 3-9.

Truax, C.B., and Mitchell, K.M. (1971). Research on certain therapist interpersonal skills in relation to process and outcome. In A. Bergin and S. Garfield (eds.), *Handbook of Psychotherapy and Behavior Change.* Wiley.

Turton, R. (1986). Bourgeois counseling and working-class clients: Some problems and practical implications. *Psychology in Society, 6,* 85-100.

van Aarde, J.A. (1987). The counseling psychologist: Professional practitioner or sociopolitical change agent. Unpublished Keynote address, SSCSA conference, Port Elizabeth.

van den Berghe, P.L. (1970). *Race and Ethnicity: Essays in Comparative Sociology.* New York: Basic Books.

van der Vyfer, J. (1976). *Seven Lectures on Human Rights.* Cape Town: Juta.

van der Vyfer, J. (1985). The bill of rights issue. *Journal for Juridical Science, 10,* 1.

van Dijk, T.A. (1987). *Communicating Racism: Ethnic Prejudice in Thought and Talk.* Newburg Park, CA: Sage.

van Dijk, T.A. (1991). *Elite Discourse and the Reproduction of Racism.* Amsterdam: University of Amsterdam.

van Dijk, T.A. (1993). *Elite Discourse and Racism.* Newbury Park, CA: Sage.

van Zyl, J. & Lasersohn, B. (1991). Introducing Michael White and his work. *SAIMFT Newsletter (Southern Transvaal Branch), 2*(1), 3-6.

Vera, H. & Feagin, J.R. (1995). African Americans' inflicted anomie. In G.E. Thomas (ed.), *Race and ethnicity in America: Meeting the challenge in the 21st century* (pp. 155-172). Washington, DC: Taylor & Francis.

Vogelman, L. (1986). Opening address to the OASSA National Conference, 17-18 May, Johannesburg.

Vogelman, L. (1987). Development of an appropriate psychology: The work of the Organisation of Appropriate Social Services in South Africa. *Psychology in Society, 7,* 24-35.

Vontress, C.E. (1969). Cultural barriers in the counseling relationship. *Personnel and Guidance* Journal, 48, 11-17.

Vontress, C.E. (1971). Racial differences: Impediments to rapport. *Journal of Counseling Psychology, 1,* 7-13.

Vontress, C.E. (1979). Cross-cultural counseling: An existential approach. *Personnel and Guidance Journal, 58,* 117-121.

Vontress, C.E. (1981). Racial and ethnic barriers in counseling. In P.B. Pedersen, J.G. Draguns, W.J. Lonner, & J.E. Trimble (eds.), *Counseling Across Cultures* (2nd ed.) (pp. 87-107). Honolulu: University of Hawaii.

Vygotsky, L.S. (1962). *Thought and Language.* New York: Wiley.

Vygotsky, L.S. (1986). *Thought and Language.* (A. Mozulin trans.) Cambridge: MIT Press (Originally published 1934).

Wade, P. & Bernstein, B.L. (1991). Culture sensitivity training and counselor's race: Effects on Black female clients' perceptions and attrition. *Journal of Counseling Psychology, 38,* 9-15.

Watkins, J.G. and Watkins, H.H. (1979-80) Ego states and hidden observers. *Journal of Altered States of Consciousness, 5* (1), 3-18.

Watkins, J.G. & Watkins, H.H. (1993). Accessing the relevant areas of maladaptive personality functioning. *American Journal of Clinical Hypnosis, 35*(4), 277-284.

Watkins, M. (1990). *Invisible Guests.* Boston, MA: Sigo Press.

Watzlawick, P. (1976). *How Real Is Real?* New York: Random House.

Watzlawick, P., Weakland, J.H., & Fisch, P. (1974). *Change: Principles of Problem Formation and Problem Resolution.* New York: Norton.

Webster, E. (1981). Servants of apartheid? In J. Rex (ed.), *Apartheid and Social Research* (pp. 85-113). Paris: Unesco.

Weigert, E. (1954). Countertransference and self-analysis of the psycho-analyst. *International Journal of Psychoanalysis, 35,* 242-246.

Welsing, F.C. (1974). Conspiracy to make Blacks inferior. *Ebony, 29,* 84-94.

Wetherell, M. & Potter, J. (1992). *Mapping the Language of Racism: Discourse and the Legitimation of Exploitation.* New York: Harvester Wheatsheaf.

Wexler, P. (1983). *Critical Social Psychology.* Boston, MA: Routledge & Kegan Paul.

Whitaker, C. (1976). A systems approach to family therapy. Unpublished transcript of presentation given for the Family Study Centre, University of Missouri, Kansas City.

White, M. (1984). Pseudo-encopresis: From avalanche to victory, from vicious to virtuous cycles. *Family Systems Medicine, 2,* 150-160.

White, M. (1986a). Negative explanation, restraint, and double description: A template for family therapy. *Family Process, 25*(2), 169-184.

White, M. (1986b). Anorexia Nervosa: A cybernetic perspective. In J. Elka-Harkary (ed.), *Eating Disorders and Family Therapy.* New York: Aspen.

White, M. (1991). Deconstruction and therapy. *Dulwich Centre Newsletter, No. 3.*

White, M. & Epston, D. (1990). *Literate Means to Therapeutic Ends.* New York: Norton.

Whittle, E.P. (1985). Review of research undertaken during the period 1981-1984. *Research Bulletin, 15,* 32-37.

Wilcocks, R.W. (1932). The poor white problem in South Africa: The report of the Carnegie Commission. In *Psychological Report.* Stellenbosch: Pro Ecclesia Drukkery.

Willie, C.V., Kramer, B.M., & Brown, B.S. (1973). *Racism and Mental Health,* University of Pittsburgh Press.

Winnicott, D. (1949). Hate in the countertransference. *International Journal of Psychoanalysis, 30,* 69-74.

Winnicott, D.W. (1960). The theory of parent-infant relationship. In *The Maturational Process and the Facilitating Environment* (pp. 39-55). New York: International Universities Press.

Winnicott, D.W. (1965). *The Maturational Processes and the Facilitating Environment.* New York: International Universities Press.

Wohl, J. (1981). Intercultural psychotherapy issues, questions, and reflections. In P. Pedersen, W. Draguns, W. Lonner & J. Trimble (eds.), *Counseling Across Cultures: Revised and Expanded Edition* (pp. 133-159). Honolulu: University of Hawaii Press.

Wong, L.M. (1994). Di(s)-secting and dis(s)-closing "Whiteness": Two tales about psychology. In K. Bhavnani & A. Phoenix (eds.), *Shifting Identities Shifting Racisms: A Feminism and Psychology Reader* (pp. 133-153). Also cited as *Feminism and Psychology, 4*(1), 133-153. London, Thousand Oaks,CA & New Delhi: Sage.

Woolgar, S. (1996). Psychology, qualitative methods, and science. In J.T.E. Richardson (ed.), *Handbook of Qualitative Research Methods for Psychology and the Social Sciences* (pp. 11-24). Leicester: BPS Books.

World Health Organization (WHO) (1977). Apartheid and mental health care. *MNE. 77,* 5.

Wortley, R. (2000). Letters to the editor: A view from South Africa. *The Psychologist, 13,* 232-233.

Wrenn, G. (1962). The culturally encapsulated counselor. *Harvard Education Review, 32,* 444-449.

Wulfsohn, D.R.W. (1988). The impact of the South African Nanny on the young child. Unpublished Ph.D. Diss. University of South Africa (UNISA).

Yardley, K. (1995). Role play. In J.A. Smith, R. Harré & L.V. Langenhove (eds.), *Rethinking Methods in Psychology* (pp. 107-122). London, Thousand Oaks, CA, & New Delhi: Sage.

Yee, A.H., Fairchild, H.H., Weizmann, F., & Wyatt, G.E. (1993). Adressing psychology's problems with race. *American Psychologist 48*(11), 1132-1140.

Yerkes, R.M. (1921). Psychological examining in the United States army. *National Academy of Science,* Memack, 15.

Young, G. (1981). Thinking seriously about crime. In Fitzgerald, M. et al. (eds.), *Crime and Society.*

Zastrow, C. (1988). What really causes psychotherapy change? *Journal of Independent Social Work, 2*(3), 5-16.

Zuk, G.H. (1971). *Family Therapy: A Triadic-Based Approach.* New York: Human Sciences Press.

Index

About the Author

MARTIN STROUS is a psychotherapist and educational psychologist based in South Africa.